OBSESSIVE COMPULSIVE DISORDER: DEBBIE'S STORY

by

Deborah Eker

Contents

Still Hanging In There: My Struggle With Obsessive Compulsive Disorder

by

Deborah Eker

Three Reasons

My story is now being written for a number of reasons. Reason one is that I would like to share the story of my lifelong struggle with obsessive compulsive disorder with others who may have the same disability or similar disabilities. I was able to diagnose myself with OCD as an adult after watching another person with the same problem. I believe that I was born with it. Reason two is to encourage anyone who has obsessive compulsive disorder to talk about it and write about it. By doing so you are acknowledging your problem and dealing with it. Talking and writing about it is therapeutic. It allows you to express your innermost feelings and thoughts as well as writing abilities. Reason three is to emphasize that a person with mental disabilities must find the right therapist who practices the right type of therapy in order to be cured.

My story as presented is told in my own unedited words. It is written episodically and not strictly chronologically because most of the events that I write about happened concurrently. The story is based on my own memories of the events that took place. Some names have been changed. Certain aspects of my life may be omitted as they may not particularly pertain to the story being told or they may not have particular interest to readers. Also persons with obsessive compulsive disorder may be in such a fog when suffering from that condition that they may either blank out or do not remember clearly events that have taken place.

What is Obsessive Compulsive Disorder?

What is obsessive compulsive disorder? My own definition is that the sufferer is missing serotonin in the brain. Serotonin is a vital component of rational thought. I was diagnosed in my thirties but I believe that I had it all my life. I have always had trouble thinking logically.

When it comes down to it, however, obsessive compulsive disorder is feeling a compulsion. Feeling that you have to do something. If you feel that you have to do something and that your whole life is revolving around that one thing, and that it is affecting how you act, feel, and think, and that it is on your mind continuously throughout the day, then that is obsessive compulsive disorder. Having these feelings can make you feel anxious, confused, disoriented, hyperactive, tired, nervous, and tense and that the only way to relieve it is to do that something that is preying on your mind. You might feel that something is in the wrong place or out of line and that you need to move it. A book may be shelved in the wrong place or is not in an even line with the other books on the shelf. You feel nervous and tense and that the only way to remove that nervous feeling and tension is to move the book to a different place or position.

Some of the most common symptoms of obsessive compulsive disorder are repeated checking, repeatedly performing an action over and over again, repeatedly saying something over and over again, keeping useless lists, mutilating yourself, impatience and rushing, clock-watching, rigidity, inappropriate sexual urges, fanaticism: believing in something to the extent that you whole life revolves around the belief, extreme cleaning and washing, and hoarding, etc.

When I was twenty-five I went to a fashion consultant who told me that the colour beige did not look good on me. On my way home all I could think of was that I had to tear off all my clothes that I was wearing and throw away everything that I owned. I felt anxious and nervous and all that I could think about was ridding myself of these clothes. When I got home that is exactly what I did. Everything that I owned went into the garbage except a top and pants that were blue and a jacket that was black. For the next few days I had to completely buy everything that I could find to replace the other clothes. A number of years later I had a purple nylon rain jacket. The jacket was a perfectly good jacket and looked nice. I, however, got it into my mind that there was something wrong with it and that it did not look good. I threw it in the garbage even though I had nothing else to replace it with.

Another example of obsessive compulsive behaviour happened recently. I know that there is a restaurant in Toronto's First Canadian Place that serves a white fish salad. This salad, served by Pumpernickel's Deli, is enormous, as is the piece of fish that tops it. The white fish is baked, with minimal sodium and cholesterol levels. On one particular day I developed a craving for the white fish. Even though it was not convenient for me to go into Toronto, and I had no reason to go in, and I also felt tired, I became obsessed with rushing in to Toronto to eat the white fish salad at Pumpernickel's. The obsession lasted for a few days and I could not think of anything else. My husband was not that excited about going in and felt that it was only for me to eat although I kept insisting that it was to look around at the stores. He said that he would go to Toronto, but go normally, not just to rush in so I could eat something. My father-in-law also requested that we go in on another day as this day would be inconvenient because there were some things we all had to do. This curbed my obsession. I realized that I did not feel like rushing into Toronto at all. I can eat the white fish salad whenever we go in at a convenient time or we go in for a definite reason. My craving for the white fish was so great that I did not realize that I was, in fact, too tired to go in that day, and that it was inconvenient for all our schedules.

This is an example from history that provides an example of a variety of obsessive compulsive disorder symptoms in a famous person. The famous political and social philosopher and theorist Karl Marx took over thirty years to write his famous work <u>Capital: A Critique of Political Economy</u> and it was still unfinished when he died in 1883. This work consisted of three volumes. The first volume was published in 1867. The second and third volume were published from unfinished notes in 1885 and 1894, respectively. He was in the British National Library in London almost every day from when it opened to when it closed writing and rewriting his work. He was meticulous about what he was writing and if the smallest new fact became known, he would rewrite everything. He would rewrite pages or paragraphs over and over again. His publisher had accepted Volume I but he did not hand it in and kept rewriting it until it was finally published. He did not work other than earn some money from newspapers articles because he was all-consumed with his writings and with the promotion of Marxism which encompassed his entire life. Karl Marx, his wife Jennie Marx, and their children had to be supported by his friend, collaborator, and fellow Marxist, Fredrick Engels, who despite his Marxist beliefs was a wealthy factory owner and lived life well while Marx and his family were almost totally dependent on Engels for financial support.

Can you see the different aspects of obsessive compulsive disorder in this example?

Often a person with obsessive compulsive disorder will feel that a piece of writing is not written properly or does not look right and will feel compelled to write it over and over again without anything really changing. If the writing is accompanied by an extreme belief in a particular philosophy this also adds to the obsession. The person will be so obsessed about this written work that the need to keep writing it takes precedence to everything else including his own well-being and the well-being of his family.

The unresolved feelings of wanting to do something can bring extreme feelings of anxiety and tension. The person with obsessive compulsive disorder will feel that they can only find relief if they give in to the compulsion. They may find temporary relief but this will not solve the problem. Obsessive compulsive disorder is a vicious cycle because if you give into one obsession or compulsion another obsession or compulsion will just replace it. It can become a never ending cycle. Obsessive compulsive disorder has to be fought. Recognizing it and wanting to fight it is ninety per cent of the battle. The other ten per cent consists of medication and intensive therapy.

The Beginning

I do not remember as much as I would like to about my childhood. Mostly I have had to be told. I was a slow eater, a slow reader, a slow writer. My thoughts were distorted. I used to spread out building blocks on the floor in my bedroom and they had to be perfectly straight. I also kept file folders and copious lists of people and things.

My parents fought constantly. My mother was always complaining that when I was born, a year after their marriage, she wasn't ready to be a mother. My younger brother came along four years after me.

Mother was always complaining that she had to stay home all day with two unappreciative brats. We did not have much disposable income because my father's salary as a credit manager was very low. I always thought that we were desperately poor, which shows how distorted my thoughts were. We always had a house and our own car. My parents just didn't buy me a lot of toys. What presents I did receive came for my birthday or good report cards.

I also took statements literally, even if they were made in anger and forgotten. My mother always insisted that she and Dad were in love when they got married, but I always thought she got married because society expected women to get married. When they fought, she and Dad went at each other tooth and nail. She used to hit him with a stick. Her anger at the least little thing made me afraid of her. I used to hide in my room and pray that they would not fight. Mother used to explain that while she was happily married, she loved a good fight and my father also loved a good fight. They were probably just kidding, but I took them literally. Mostly they fought over us children. All that children ever do is to ask, ask, ask for her to do things and give nothing in return. She was always threatening to leave her marriage and leave us alone to fend for ourselves. I believe that the guilt trips she placed on me may have triggered the obsessive compulsive disorder.

It was when I started school that my obsessive compulsive disorder symptoms first manifested themselves to a worrisome degree. I read and wrote very slowly to the point where I could not complete classroom tests. I was unable to properly organize my desk at school or my homework. My lack of organizational skills persisted into my high school and university years, with disastrous results. I giggled in inappropriate situations and I could not sit still in class. I was unable to focus on what I had to do in school and was always asking classmates and teachers to help me.

I have a cousin, G.K., who is a well-known children's author living in New York. He wrote his first book at the age of twelve, as a Grade 7 homework writing assignment. His book was so good that my aunt, who is my mother's sister, Gertrude, successfully submitted the book to a publisher. G.K. has been writing ever since.

My mother, Stella, recently said to me on the telephone, "Debbie, you should have been a writer yourself, living in New York City".

To which I answered, "It is your fault, mother, that I did not. I could write and wanted to write as soon as I was able to put pen to paper. You never encouraged me. In fact you neglected me."

I was a child prodigy, but apparently my parents did not notice that even though it was obvious. Here is my story.

My Family

My father, Maurice Peterson, was born in Montreal. His parents were Samuel Peterson and Elizabeth Strachan, who were both born in the Ukraine. My mother, Stella Samuels, was also born in Montreal. Her parents were Geoffrey Samuels and Clara Simons, who were both born in Montreal. My mother always criticized my father's parents as being uncultured immigrants while her parents were born in Canada. This view was somewhat distorted as her parents were only first generation Canadians and her grandparents were born in Lithuania and Romania.

My paternal grandfather, Samuel Peterson, worked in clothing stores all his life. He was very intelligent and liked to read Russian classical literature. If he had been an educated man he might have been a teacher or a librarian. My maternal grandmother, Elizabeth Strachan, had finished school in the Ukraine and also liked reading classical literature. My maternal grandfather, Geoffrey Samuels, and his brothers owned an electrical parts business Electicon. The company was mismanaged and it went out of business. It failed to accept a buyout offer from Berelli Tires because the oldest brother, Carl Samuels, did not want to deal with Italians. A poor business decision and a rather prejudiced outlook towards others, as I see it. After this happened, my grandfather got a job as a salesman. He and my grandmother, Clara, thought that an education was unimportant and that it was more important to be "a good person". They never praised me for being smart or doing well in school.

My father was the elder of two brothers. I believe that he had undetected obsessive compulsive disorder. He was highly intelligent and an omnivorous reader. But he was totally ambitious and unable to discipline himself for study at the university level. His failure at education gave him an inferiority complex. He went to McGill University for one year but failed and never went back. He then got a job as a cashier in a television store.

My mother is the elder of two sisters. I also believe that she had obsessive compulsive disorder that she does not want to admit to. She is very rigid in her ideas and the way she does things. Everything from the way people look and behave and to the way things appear and are placed has to be what she terms "good" or "perfect". When I have asked her what she means by "good" or "perfect" she is unable to give a clear definition and simply says that she likes "good people" or "perfect people" and that she "likes things to be good" and likes "likes things to be perfect". She always has said that she wants to meet people and have friends just like her. She also has an ethnic complex. She wants her friends to be from the same ethnic group that we are from. This is a foolish and restrictive idea that has resulted in the fact that at the present she has few friends.

My mother went to McGill University for one year but dropped out because she did not want to study.

She then went and trained as a laboratory technician at a Montreal hospital. She worked as a laboratory technician for about four or five years in at Montreal hospitals.

In a recent telephone conversation with me, my mother admitted, "When I dropped out of McGill University, I didn't know what I wanted out of life. I did not want to study. I just wanted to get married and have children. Once I had two children, I could not go back in time."

"Why were you always accusing Bradley and me of not appreciating what you did for us?" I asked. "All that I ever heard during my growing up years was that we should thank you and Daddy for sacrificing what you really wanted out of life in order to bring us up. We did not ask to be born. You wanted to have us. It isn't fair."

My mother answered, "At the time that you and Bradley were born, I was forced to have children. Women who were good people got married and had children. I had no way of knowing how much work was involved in bringing up two children."

"That was your problem," I protested. "Just because you were too lazy to do research and find out what having children would involve, you had no right to expect us to appreciate us being born and brought up. You are rationalizing you treatment of us, that is all you were doing.'

In answer, my mother got upset. "I have nobody to talk to," she cried. "Your father died and left me. You and Bradley are no use to me. Since your father died, I have nobody to talk to."

My mother doesn't understand that her mistreatment of my father killed him at age 56 and that her mistreatment of me and Bradley turned us away from her. She does not realize that she, herself, ruined her own life.

When I was born in Montreal, my father, Maurice, was earning a very low salary as a cashier in a store. My mother, Stella, was working as a laboratory technologist. My mother had to stop working to raise me and later my brother because she could not afford daycare or a sitter. With the loss of my mother's income, our family had to live on my father's very low salary. For my mother, this was an enormous adjustment, one that she did not like. At the age of 24, my mother was not ready to be a mother.

In a recent conversation with me, my mother told me, "I did not know what having a baby would involve. I went through my pregnancy, literally blindfolded. By the time I did find out what was involved, it was too late, I could not give the baby back." What type of insane person wants to give back her own flesh and blood?

When I was eighteen months old, my Aunt Gertrude, who was not yet married, won a teddy bear shooting darts at Belmont Park. Naturally, I was given the teddy bear to play with. I named the bear, Elvis, which surprised both of my parents. There was nobody named Elvis in my family and my parents did not know anybody named Elvis. That an eighteen month old baby was aware of the name Elvis, probably because she had seen Elvis Presley on television, made no impression on my mother.

What made an impression on my mother was that my father, Maurice, was a ferocious talker and very interested in law. On her knees, she begged Morris to go to university to study law. As a lawyer he could earn a better salary than what he was earning as a cashier. But Maurice refused. He said, "It is too late for me to return to university. It'll be too hard. I have a wife and a child." My mother took his refusal very badly.

Unlike Stella, Maurice was ready to be a parent. He loved me very much. But my mother was always putting him down, so I did not value his love. I did think that my mother did not love me.

When I was two, I began asking my mother for toys. My mother said to me, "You must never ask for things because it isn't nice to ask for things. We are poor because you father does not make a good living. We had you a year after our wedding, so we have very little money. If we had not had you so soon, I would have been able to keep working and I might have saved more money. If you father would go back for law, we would be rich and I could buy you lots of toys. But because Daddy won't go back to university and study we are poor."

When I was three, I began asking my two sets of grandparents, maternal and paternal, questions about the family history. Both grandmothers showed me pictures of relatives. That it was unusual for a three year old to ask questions about genealogy before the subject became commonplace escaped my mother. My father was impressed with my questions. My mother ignored the whole thing.

What my mother did do was nag my father about our perceived poverty stricken situation. My father did not take my mother's nagging silently but fought back.

When I was four, my maternal grandparents bought a duplex in the Cote St. Luc area of Montreal that my family would share with my maternal aunt and new uncle, Gertrude and Isadore K. The duplex was spacious. Each flat was identical with large bedrooms, a kitchen, living room, and dining room. A vestibule was at the entrance to the first floor and a flight of stairs led up to the second storey. The duplex was semi-detached and enjoyed spacious front and back lawns. We occupied the bottom flat and my aunt and uncle and soon their son, G., occupied the top flat. The master bedroom had an ensuite bathroom and my new baby brother, Bradley, and I shared a large bathroom.

Reminiscing about our Cote St. Luc home in a recent conversation we had, my mother said, "It was not the right house for us. We wanted to buy one of the duplexes on the side streets but by the time we were able to buy, the side street duplexes were sold out, so we had to buy on the main drag."

"So why did we move in?" I asked.

My mother answered, "Both of our families wanted to buy a house and the cheapest way to do that was to buy a duplex. You know, when Dad and I got married, we could have bought a bungalow in the older section of Cote St. Luc for $12,000. It would have been a struggle carrying a bungalow on one salary, but Grandfather Geoffrey would have helped us with a down payment. At the time we thought we could not afford a bungalow, but looking back we should have found the money somewhere. We would have had a nice bungalow on a quiet side street, instead of a duplex on a busy main street."

My mother gave birth to my brother, Bradley, when we first moved in. At first it seemed that all was going well with our family but problems soon developed. Having another baby meant that my father's salary supported a family of four. By now he had become a credit manager through a correspondence course, but his salary remained low. My mother felt she could not return to work because having her two children cared for by either a grandmother or a babysitter was "not the right thing to do." Instead of going to work she nagged my father that she "was stuck in all day with her two demanding brats."

"Other wives get a break from their children once in a while," she screamed, "only I am tied down like a dog."

My father answered, "And other wives don't nag their husbands because they are not millionaires."

My mother saw that other women in Cote St. Luc were married to rich professional husbands. Because her husband was a lowly credit manager she had an enormous inferiority complex. The other wives went to work and left their children with housekeepers. My mother could not afford to hire a housekeeper and would have had to rely on her mother.

She degraded my father to us two children. 'Your father is a good man," she said, "but he is only a credit manager. He would be a better person if he had become a lawyer."

To my father she said, "You have as many brains as the rich men who live around here. Why can't you force yourself to go back for law instead of insisting on being a credit manager?"

To add insult to injury, I was unable to make friends with the other girls in the neighbourhood because they were rich and I was not. I acquired my mother's inferiority complex. Not all of the families in the neighbourhood were rich, but the less affluent families did not have immigrant grandparents as I did. My father did not mind my associating with poorer children. He said, "Sometimes children from poorer homes are nicer than children from affluent homes." I was able to make friends with some of the poorer children.

My early childhood was scarred by my parents' fighting. I was afraid of their fighting and decided that I would be a "good little girl" and did not disturb my mother unduly, so that she would not fight with my father. This did not help.

Maternal Family Education and Values

"I wanted to be married, but I didn't want to take crap from my husband," said my mother in a recent conservation that I had with her. "I wanted to be-you-know-assertive. I wanted to have children, but I wanted my children to appreciate what I did for them." With these words, my mother all but admitted that she got married and had children because she could not face the stigma of being a single, childless woman in Montreal.

Certainly my mother had a very conservative upbringing in Montreal. She always considered that she had a liberal upbringing. That is because my maternal grandparents, George Samuels and Clara Simons, were born in Montreal, and although they were Jewish, they were very unreligious. While other Jewish families in the Montreal of the 1930's and 1940's were keeping kosher and running to synagogues, my grandparents took my mother and her sister, my aunt Gertrude, on shopping and theater excursions to New York City.

But the Jewish community in Montreal in those days was very, very, conservative. Not just the Jewish community but everybody in the entire province of Quebec was backwards. All Anglophones including Jews, attended The Protestant School board of Greater Montreal. The Protestant School Board believed sternly in one mantra: Be a good person. And being a good person meant doing the right thing to do at all times. If doing the right thing clashed with the requirements of earning a good living or merely surviving, then so be it. at least you would die knowing that you were a good person. These ideas still persisted many decades later after I was born and when I went to school in Montreal.

My maternal grandparents and my great-aunt and uncles, who were their siblings swallowed this mantra hook, line, and sinker. One of my great-aunts, Esther Samuels, got married in her late thirties to Holden Adams, who was a survivor of the Nazi concentration camps. My Canadian-born great-aunts and great-uncles hated Holden because he had done bad things in order to stay alive.

One of my great-uncles, Johnny Samuels, once said, "Holden is a despicable person because of the things he did to escape the concentration camps. I would never have done those bad things. I would have died in the concentration camps, rather than do what he did."

I asked Uncle Johnny, "What purpose would it serve to die? Hideous atrocities were done to the Jews by the Nazis. The one who survived had the strength of character to come to Canada and rebuild their lives."

Whereupon Johnny answered, "I would rather have died because I would rather have had the satisfaction of knowing that I was a good person."

Balderdash! But my grandparents believed this. They passed it on to my mother. My mother lived by a puritanical moral code. for her, being a good person meant getting married and having two children.

My mother did well in school and got into McGill University, but she dropped out of McGill after her first year. She told me, "I discovered that to succeed in university I would have to study very hard. I did not want to study. I wanted to have fun and run to New York. I also wanted to get married and have children. I was afraid that if I was too smart and too well-educated I would never get married."

Not only my grandparents, but all of their siblings were appallingly ignorant. My great-grandparents on my maternal grandfather's side immigrated to Canada from Lithuania, which at the end of the nineteenth century was part of Czarist Russia's Pale of Settlement. Jews who lived in this area were not allowed to attend school. Now, I am certain that other Lithuanian Jewish immigrants were eager to send their children to school in Canada, especially because in Canada all parents were required to send their children to school. Not so, my great-grandfather, Cyril Samuels sent his children to school only to learn the basics of reading and writing and arithmetic. He took all of his seven sons, including my grandfather, out of school after grade six, to work in his parts business. His three daughters, my great aunts, Ruth, Patsy, and Esther were forced to stay home and vegetate. Cyril expected that they would get married and that their husbands would support them.

All my life, I have been ashamed of my grandfather's ignorance. My mother insists that my grandfather was not ignorant, he "just did not go to school. He was not ignorant, he was a good person."

My mother went on to say, "My great grandfather, Cyril Samuels came from an area in Russia where Jews were not allowed to go to school, so education was not important in his mind. In Quebec, when he and his wife Grace Samuels came over, education was not compulsory. Catholic schools were free, because the teachers were all nuns and priests but the Protestant School board was not free. They charged fees. Cyril could not afford the fees, so he did not send his children to school."

My maternal grandmother, Clara Simons, was also uneducated. Clara's father Bart Simons, was actually a wealthy Romanian immigrant restaurant owner. But Bart did not believe in education for girls, only for boys. Bart and his wife Sandra, had four children, including, my grandmother, Clara and her sister Deidre. Clara and Deidre both left school, even though their father could afford it, because they were not encouraged, as girls, to stay in school.

Neither my grandfather Geoffrey nor my grandmother Clara, believed in education. They believed that it was important to be a good person and to do good in in the world. Even though my mother and Aunt Gertrude, both did well in school, they were not praised for their educational achievements. Aunt Gertrude, was a very clever girl who did well in school, was a talented writer and poet, and completed a B.A. at Sir George Williams College. Both girls were brought up to get married, have children, and be supported by their husbands.

I did well in school and so did my brother, Bradley. But we were never praised. My mother lived by a very strong moral code which excluded educational prowess. She instilled this moral code in us. Even though she expected both Bradley and me to go to university, what we would take in university and do for a living was never discussed. Rather, she discussed the importance with us of being good people, of getting married and having children, and of always doing the right thing. For her, the most important aspect of our lives was to be dutiful children who appreciated what our parents did for us and to idolize our grandparents, who were perfect.

"You would have to go very far to find better and finer people than your grandparents," my mother said. "I want you two kids to appreciate your heritage."

"But we are both good in school, and you never praise us for being good min school," I protested.

"Why don't you praise Bradley and me for being good students?"

"In our family, we don't believe in praising children for being intelligent and being good in school," my mother answered. "It is a foregone conclusion that Jewish children are smart and will do well in school. If we praise you two children, you will get swelled heads and be conceited and you will cease to be good children. If we tell you that you are smart, you will think you are better than children who are not so smart and do not do well in school. You have to learn to be good people and to do good in the world. Lots of highly educated people are bad people who do not know the right thing to do. You children will be good children and always know the right thing to do."

Incidentally, elementary education was not compulsory in Quebec until long after it was compulsory in other parts of Canada. We did not have a provincial Ministry of Education until the 1960's. Up until then, education was in the hands of the individual Protestant and Catholic School Boards. High school was not compulsory until the 1970's.

Both of my maternal grandparents idolized the British Royal Family. My grandmother, Clara, adored both King George VI and Queen Elizabeth, particularly because of their heroic behaviour during World War II. My grandparents brought up my mother and Aunt Gertrude to emulate Queen Elizabeth II and Princess Margaret. In their combined view, the two generations of the Royal Family were good people who did the right thing. Queen Elizabeth in particular was a good person who did her duty and married Prince Philip. Margaret was also a good person who "did her duty" and bowed to her family's wishes that she not marry Peter Townsend.

My mother swallowed her parents' values without ever thinking about whether the values of the Depression Era and the Second World War applied to her own life in the 1950's. Actually, without getting into a sociological analysis, I can safely say that World War II opened new opportunities for everybody around the world who joined the armed forces and who did war work in their respective countries. It led to the development of new technologies and opened up work opportunities for women who would normally have been at home. Despite these opportunities, my grandparents stayed in the same rigid rut that the hardships of the Depression Era had forced upon them. My mother was a very conventional Jewish woman who followed her mother's path because during the 1950's and 1960's women and men were expected to marry and have children. She did not think that she had a choice.

"I had a beautiful mother who believed in the right thing to do," my mother said, "so I followed her completely. When I got married, Queen Elizabeth set the standard for all women. Of course, I copied her."

"Our family may not be educated," she continued, "but we are still an eminent family. Grandfather Geoffrey was the first Jewish Grand

Master of the Masonic Temple in Quebec, and Grandmother Clara was the first Jewish President of the Eastern Star in Quebec. When other fancy educated Jewish families were nobody, your grandparents went to Ottawa to meet the Queen and Prince Philip. They also met the Governor-General, George P. Vanier and his wife. How many educated Jewish families can boast about that? When other Jewish grandparents were keeping kosher and running to synagogues, your grandparents read all of the books written by Winston Churchill. Education enhances you but it isn't everything." My own opinion is that none of this stuff that my mother told me about my grandparents is any big deal.

Education may not be everything, but it gives you the tools to recognize lucrative business opportunities when you see them. Great grandfather Cyril, grandfather Geoffrey, and the other brothers owned an electrical parts business. They could have gotten beautiful government contracts to supply both the war effort and the home front, particularly since domestic manufacturing had to be curtailed in favour of the war effort. Their lack of education caused them not to have the business knowledge to pursue this area which could have given the business millions of dollars and provided work for hundreds and possibly thousands of people. Worse than that, for my morally stern grandfather, making money out of a war was not the right thing to do. He did not seem to understand that the government needed electrical parts supplied for the war and that by doing this and providing employment he would be helping the Allies in the war effort.

After the war when there was a shortage of domestic building materials, Cyril and his sons donated free of charge, building materials for a new building for their synagogue. The business, however, needed money, and they could have made money out of this construction project, but they did not charge the synagogue because that was not the right thing to do. Giving away business resources crippled the business which was already not doing well. They had a buyout offer from another company but one of the brothers did not want to sell. Rather than offend him they did not take the buyout offer and as a result the business went bankrupt.

Obsessive Compulsive Disorder Begins

It was around this time that symptoms of obsessive compulsive disorder were really apparent in me. I could dress and feed myself, but completed tasks slowly, too slowly. I was also very confused about my surroundings and made up stories. I also giggled in inappropriate situations. When I arranged building blocks on the bedroom floor they all had to be in a straight line. I was also, as my Aunt Gertrude told me in a recent conversation "totally unobservant". She said, "When your mother was pregnant with Bradley, I never once heard you say, 'Mommy is getting fat.' When I was pregnant with G., you were seven and a half years old but you never once said, 'Auntie Gertrude is getting fat'."

Obsessive compulsive disorder was unknown in those days. All the family thought that I would outgrow the "bad habits" and get better as I matured. My mother, however, instead of trying to be supportive, started criticizing me heavily. She would say, "You just make up stories just like your grandmother." She would accuse me of being like my paternal grandmother Betty whom she did not like.

Now a small child is dependent on her parents. My mother disliked having a dependent child. She said to me, "All you do is eat and sleep and defecate. I have to work like a dog to bring you up. You have to learn to appreciate what I do for you. When I buy you food and clothes, you have to remember that they cost money and treat them with respect."

This attitude left me feeling guilty whenever my mother "did something" for me. When I misbehaved and had to be disciplined, my mother snarled at me, "We work like dogs for your upkeep and this is the thanks we get! You should be ashamed of yourself."

I started kindergarten when I was five. It was about this time that I found my interest in music. A grand piano was in my family's living room. Both my mother and my aunt played the piano. I was able to climb up on the piano bench and sit beside my mother on it. After about a week of this I asked my mother to show me how to play. My obsessive compulsive disorder made my attention span very short. My mother was skeptical of my interest in the piano because I was constantly distracted. But I persisted and finally learned how to play simple music. I also began to take piano lessons in elementary school but was too distracted to practice.

At the age of six I began to write. I was learning how to read and write in elementary school. Because my father read to Bradley and me, and told us his own stories during our pre-school years, I was already reading and enjoying books immensely. Not only was I reading simple children's stories, but also serious fiction and nonfiction. I wanted to write like the authors. I wanted to share the author's agony and I could feel her pleasure. I could also imagine her triumphs.

So I started writing myself. I wanted to write about famous people, like the President of the United States, famous singers, and royalty. My youth prevented me from doing the necessary research to establish the accuracy of what I wrote and living in Montreal I had no access to the research facilities that doing original research required. I was old enough to put good sentences together and I liked writing big words. My elementary school teachers encouraged me to write compositions and from grade three onwards, our school principal wanted all of the children to have pen pals so that we could practice our writing.

At the age of ten, I wrote to a pen pal service in the United States and met a Swedish pen pal. We corresponded with each other for many years until I was in university. My pen pal, Maud, always looked forward to my letters because she said at one point, that "I wrote stories so good."

I went to summer camp from the age of nine until I was fifteen. My bunk mates liked reading my descriptive letters to my parents and my aunt and uncle. Believe it or not, when everybody at my camp wanted to write a fan letter to Ringo Starr, of the Beatles fame, who also became an actor and singer on his own, I was chosen to write it. When we were supposed to be napping after lunch, I wrote fictional stories.

Why did I not publish as a child? I did not find out why until my cousin, G., published his first novel at the age of twelve, about a bunch of schoolboys fooling around. Aunt Gertrude said, "You and I, Debbie, could not publish because we liked writing historical fiction which takes too long to research and write. Here G. wrote a simple book about a few boys."

Neither of my parents encouraged me to write. In the Quebec school system, excellence in math and science were necessary in order to pass the high school matriculations. To excel in math and science requires a rational thinking process. Because of my obsessive compulsive disorder, rational thought was impossible during my school years. Therefore I could not grasp either math or science. My bad performances in math and science worried the same teachers who encouraged me to write. "You will have to forget about your writing ability and concentrate on your math and science," my grade six teacher told me, "otherwise you will fail your high school matriculations."

During my school years, other symptoms of obsessive compulsive disorder manifested themselves in me. I was teased and made fun of a lot by my classmates, which made me cry. I also wrote and read very slowly, consequently failing tests. At the same time I boasted about excellence in English and history so that my classmates accused me of bragging. The obsessive compulsive disorder produced personality traits in me that made it impossible for me to make friends.

It was the educational system in Montreal that brought out my major obsessive compulsive disorder symptoms and these started when I was in elementary school. Because I was very slow, I could not complete tests. Rational thought is required to excel in math and science. I could not grasp either, because, thanks to my obsessive compulsive disorder, I was incapable of rational thought. Where I did succeed at a level beyond my years was in reading, writing, English, geography, history, and politics. I was an avid reader of books beyond my years and also began writing little short stories. This same learning process extended into my high school years in Montreal and in Toronto where my family moved after I graduated from high school in Montreal and where I attended Grade 13. My parents, however, especially my mother, never praised me for my intellectual prowess. They told me that to graduate school I needed to be good in math and science. Throughout both elementary and high school I did not have many friends because my obsessive compulsive disorder symptoms gave people the wrong impression of me.

Be A Good Person

I found the rigid formality of the Protestant School Board of Greater Montreal oppressive. Throughout my school years, teachers and textbooks exhorted us to do the "right thing to do", when even though what they considered "right" clashed with the requirements of earning a living. I felt that they were telling us that "it was better to be a good person who was poor than a rich person who was not a good person".

Both my parents and my maternal grandparents strongly believed in the "right thing to do" and all exhorted me to be "a good person". Throughout my growing up years, I heard from my mother, 'Nothing is as important as being a good person. A good person does not want to do well in school or make a lot of money. A good person only wants to do good in the world. It is better to be on welfare and be a good person than to work and be a bad person." My mother always emphasized, "the right thing to do". All this was rather strange considering my mother was always nagging my father about how much money he made and that she was unable to explain what "the right thing to do" actually meant. So I grew up with these ideas emphasized at both school and at home.

My parents stressed the importance of being dutiful to your family as the most important component of being a good person. In a recent conversation that I had with my mother, she said, "I don't know why people have to spill their guts out about their family in a memoir. If you don't like the way your parents treated you, be different. If a person's father sexually abused them they should just marry somebody not like him. Either way you forget about it and keep going." I had been telling my mother about Viga Boland's recent memoir of her sexual abuse by her father, <u>No Tears For My Father</u>, which my mother totally disagrees with. My mother does not understand why people want to write memoirs of their lives. She thinks everything should be private.

Ever so reluctantly, I de-emphasized writing, history, and English, and concentrated on math and science. I still had trouble with both subjects. Whenever I complained to my mother about any trouble I was having in school, she yelled at me, "That should be the least problem you have. I don't want to hear about your problems. I have my own. I'm the one who has to make ends meet on your father's low salary. Leave me alone." Through sheer tenacity, I did pass the math and science matriculations. I graduated from high school in Montreal with honours in English, French, and history. But I also resolved never to bother my mother again.

My mother was reluctant to go to work, even though she had a career, and Bradley and I were in school all day. She justified it was the same familiar refrain about "The right thing to do."

From Montreal to Toronto

Aunt Gertrude and Uncle Isadore moved to Toronto prior to my finishing high school. He was working for an accounting firm in Montreal and training to be a chartered accountant. After he graduated he got a job in Toronto.

After I graduated from high school in Montreal my family moved to Toronto. We moved to Toronto because my father lost his job as a credit manager in Montreal. He got a new job as a credit manager at Copp Clark, a book publisher, in Toronto. We first lived in a rental flat at Wilmington and Finch and then moved to our own house at Don Mills and McNicoll. My mother returned to work. She was able to get a job as a laboratory technologist in a hospital. But far from contenting her, the job left her seething with rage. Part of the reason for this was that she had to work shifts. The other part was that she felt she had to work and run a home which for her constituted two jobs. My father only did one job, as far as she was concerned. Everyday either before work or in the evening she cleaned the house from top to bottom.

I helped her with the family meals, but did not see the need for my mother's fanatical housecleaning. When I did the laundry, she complained that I ruined her work uniforms.

"Everybody at work irons their uniforms." she cried. "I can't iron them because I am too tired. I have to work and run a boarding house and it isn't fair."

I should mention at this point that my father was an omnivorous reader, but he was totally useless at working with his hands. That he would not try to work with his hands irritated my mother. My father could not change a lightbulb. My mother blamed my paternal grandparents for my father's mechanical ineptitude. "His parents never owned a house", she complained to Barry and me, "They always rented apartments. They never taught him to be handy with his hands. But now that he has his own home, your father should try to work with his hands."

To my father she constantly complained that she saw other men in the libraries borrow books on home improvement while he did not. "When I see what other men do, and you don't do, I get angry and angrier." she yelled at him.

My father agreed with me that the house did not need a daily complete cleaning. My mother raged at him for not doing as much cleaning as she wanted him to. "I can't work shifts and clean the house," she complained. "Anybody else would die if his wife had to work as hard as I do. You are a lazy selfish pig." Well one day this happened. My father, who had diabetes, but was not taking care of himself, died. My father had been diagnosed with diabetes by his doctor Irving Zelcer but had not been told to take insulin. He also continued to smoke and did not eat right. Sometimes I think that he just gave up due to the fighting with my mother. He died during the period I was employed in a serious of disastrous secretarial jobs.

Grade 13

I enrolled in Grade 13 at MacKenzie Collegiate in Toronto. Here I was able to drop math and science and concentrate on English and history. But in the Toronto high school the teachers told me that the format for writing fiction was inappropriate to academic writing. Academic writing was how I had to write all my essays in Grade 13 and in university if I was to go there. I recently told my husband, Glen, that "academic writing with its stiff formality destroyed my writing style." I still exhibited obsessive compulsive disorder symptoms in high school in Toronto but was at least able to make friends better than when I was at high school in Montreal.

My two English teachers in Grade 13 applauded my fictional writing style. One of my English courses was "Women in Literature". One of the books that we studied was St. Joan by George Bernard Shaw. My teacher in that course read my essay on St. Joan to the class because she liked it so much.

"Debbie", she said, "has the right idea on how to write. Here is how she began her story. Joan of Arc...", That being said, I would really like to understand the thought process that led me to specialize in political science at York University, where I decided to study after graduating from Grade 13. But I think I now do understand. My father was involved in the Liberal Party of Canada and did volunteer work for them. He used to take me from the time I was a small child to their meetings and rallies and wanted me to have a career in politics when I grew up. My mother was totally unsupportive. "Mother wanted me to concentrate on making a living and forget about politics. I wasn't going to argue with her." My father told me. She said to my father, "If you wanted a political career you should have gone for law."

Although as I previously said, my father did not want to go back to university to be a lawyer, he wanted me to go for law and said that I would make a terrific lawyer. My mother told him that he was just trying to live vicariously through me. I, however, had no interest in taking law in university. I did not know what I wanted to study and what career to educate myself for.

York University

So after graduating from high school I decided to study political science at York University because I had an interest in it. I had, however, no idea about what I would do with it. I did not take English or history because I was afraid that the only career avenue available to English and history graduates was teaching and I could not face being in front of a class. In university I felt that the pressure of writing exams "set my brain on fire". Reading abstract theory and statistics exacerbated my obsessive compulsive disorder symptoms. To ease my pain I worked as a student reporter for the university newspaper Excalibur. Just as I had the ability for writing fiction, I was able to go around the campus and cover events, writing news articles for the paper. I found that I enjoyed newspaper reporting more than my studies and my marks suffered.

I wrote twenty-six articles for the newspaper. I also was able to make some friends at the university. My marks, however, suffered and I was only able to graduate with a three year degree in political science.

During these first three years at York when I reported on Campus news for the university newspaper, Excalibur, although I enjoyed writing very much, I ran into conflict because of my political views. Although I was brought up in a politically liberal family, as an undergraduate student, I turned away from those liberal views to more conservative views. My conservative views set me at loggerheads with the other Excalibur student reporters who were politically left wing, both at the federal and provincial levels. Here again my obsessive compulsive disorder affected my behaviour. I had a chance to make friends with a group of very nice people, and blew this chance by verbally fighting with them over differing viewpoints.

Before I started my third year at university, I told my mother that "York University had a creative writing program." My mother was shocked, "Why aren't you in it? she asked me. "Because I didn't know about it.", I answered. My mother was angry. "We brought you up with proper values." she said to me. "It is up to you to find out about your own university studies. It isn't up to me to find you a career." Upon consulting the university calendar I discovered that the Faculty of Fine Arts' creative writing program was by special selection and to be admitted to it a student had to submit a portfolio of fictional writing that had been published. I had none and so was not eligible. Instead, since I wanted to write and be a journalist I took in my third year Contemporary Canadian Journalism and The Mass Media in Canada.

During these three years at York I did not fare too well with my professors. My obsessive compulsive disorder caused me to be very argumentative and opinionated. If I disagreed with them about what they said and if I had to see them with questions about essays I was very abrupt and rude to them.

In writing essays, I had to use as a template, an essay handbook that was popular in universities. Essays written according to this formula had to be very structured and formal. Not even in MacKenzie Collegiate during Grade 13 had I been forced to write this way. Being a lover of fiction I found this style very difficult to master. Consequently, I panicked at writing essays this way. I also received low marks on them such as C and C+. On the other hand exams had been the lifeblood of my elementary and high school years, so I did better on exams. Even so, my marks were low, because exams were not a major component of the courses that I took.

I remember that my professors knew that I was a reporter for <u>Excalibur</u>. At least one of them told me that writing for news stories was inappropriate to academic writing. I did not listen to them.

York University had an academic workshop to teach student essay writing. Although one third year professor asked me to go to the writing workshop, I rudely refused. My writing style was good enough for MacKenzie Collegiate, so it was bloody well good enough for York University. At least, that is what my distorted thought was at the time. A second third year professor accused me of being very rude to his secretary and to him when I yelled at him, "Essay writing in this university can destroy a person's writing talent." In my distorted thinking I felt that the professors were all against me and trying to destroy my talent as a writer. This is what obsessive compulsive disorder can do to you. I can make your thinking about sometime so rigid that no one else's opinion matters can even be considered.

Although I had made a few friends in Grade 13 and at York University through Excalibur my friendships did not last. Because of my obsessive compulsive disorder symptoms, my friends complained that I was immature, and they deserted me.

Summer Jobs

In the three summers after each of my three years at York University I worked for the Ministry of the Attorney-General as a clerk-typist for the Supreme Court of Ontario and at the York County Court House. My uncle, Steven Peterson, was a senior civil servant for the Ministry of the Treasury and Intergovernmental Affairs and he was able to get me the summer jobs. I don't remember much about the jobs or how I performed but if my obsessive compulsive disorder affected it they either did not notice or did not care because I was only a summer student.

Trying For Journalism School

I enjoyed reporting for Excalibur so much that reporting superseded studying and essays. If a career as a writer was closed to me because I had never had any fiction published, a career in journalism was the next best thing. During my time as a reporter for Excalibur I wrote 26 articles. So I had a portfolio to show any journalism school that I applied to.

Ryerson University offered two journalism programs. One that was three years long for students who had graduated high school, and one that was two years long for university graduates. I applied to this program during my third year at York.

To be admitted to the two year program, an applicant had to present him or herself for an interview with Richard Lumn, the Journalism Department Chair and with Marq de Villiers, the two year program instructor.

I think that my obsessive compulsive disorder symptoms may have affected my performance at the interview. Both Lumn and de Villiers told me after the interview that I had done well. But rather than accepting me to the two year program, they put me on a waiting list. They thought that I was a good candidate for the program, but that they had found "better" candidates. I would be admitted to the program if one of the "better" candidates did not respond affirmatively to the offer of acceptance. I was also free to re-apply.

I did re-apply, at a later date, during my therapy with Helen Sugar. Because secretarial jobs had not worked out, I tried again journalism at Ryerson University, in their two-year program. This time the interview was a disaster, probably because of my obsessive compulsive disorder symptoms, and I was not admitted to the program.

Carleton University in Ottawa has always had a four-year journalism program for high school graduates, and a one year Honours Bachelor of Journalism Degree for graduates of a three year university program. I applied to the one year Honours Program. I was rejected. Carleton University's Faculty of Journalism believed that because of my mediocre marks, I did not have the ability to complete an Honours Bachelor's Degree.

They did offer me a ray of hope. The Faculty of Journalism stipulated that for mature students, they could overlook my mediocre marks if I successfully completed one year of employment on a newspaper. I was invited to re-apply after one year of employment.

Me As A Reporter

I found an ad in the <u>Toronto Star</u> for a reporting job on a community newspaper in northern Ontario, in the Town of Iroquois Falls, located near Timmins. There the local paper was called <u>The Enterprise</u> which was a weekly publication. I applied for the job, but I lost it after three months, largely due to my obsessive compulsive disorder symptoms but also due to internal newspaper factors that I shall explain further on. I enjoyed reporting and taking photographs. But again my obsessive compulsive disorder resulted in inappropriate behaviour on my part. In addition to my other symptoms, I now did a lot of checking on already completed tasks, and a lot of verbal repetition.

The other reasons why I lost the job were due to the Publisher, William C. Cavell. In Iroquois Falls, he was a prominent figure known by everybody. He had one full-time editor, Mrs. Albert Hall, who, doubled as a reporter. Cavell hired an extra reporter between October and February each year to cover holiday festivities. He would fire this extra reporter in February of the New Year. I was this extra reporter who was hired for the Christmas season and then fired.

Looking back on my failure in Iroquois Falls, my mother said to me, in a recent telephone conversation, "Your failure was because of Daddy and me. We naively let you take a job that had no future. At the time, Daddy was working for Copp Clark, whose textbooks were ordered by the Iroquois Falls Board of Education. Daddy knew the school board administrator, a woman named Bertha. Daddy could have telephoned Bertha and found out that Cavell was locally known as "Hire'em and Fire'em Bill." You could then have not even applied for the Christmas job. If you had continued answering ads for newspaper reporter jobs, instead of grabbing the first one, you might have gotten a better job on a better newspaper. You might have had a successful reporting career for a few years, not just one, and you might have made it to Carleton University with that work experience behind you."

I was there only a short time, between October and February, and did reporting, writing, and taking photographs. I had thirty-nine articles and photographs published in this newspaper.

I came home from Iroquois Falls absolutely not knowing what to do for a career. By now my parents had bought a house at Don Mills and McNicoll. Bradley was now at the University of Waterloo studying Electrical engineering and participating in their co-operative study and work programme.

I have since found out that I could also have applied to community colleges such as Mohawk College, here in Hamilton, which has a journalism program or to Humber College's School of Journalism, instead of putting all admission applications into two universities.

My husband, Glen, said recently, "You could have gone on to the University of Western Ontario's School of Journalism after you completed your fourth year of political science at York University if you had persisted with your goal of a journalism degree. But instead you were seduced by the University of Toronto, a big-name university with their flashy Graduate School of Library Science. Despite your obsessive compulsive disorder symptoms, you might have gotten a full-time reporting job if you had done graduate work at Western in Journalism. A Library Science Master's Degree is an easy graduate degree, nothing more. It was always hard to get a full-time job in a library, even with U of T's M.L.S."

"If when you were originally at York, you had known about the graduate journalism degree at Western, you might have been focussed towards an Honours B.A. and had the marks to get into Western's journalism program after you graduated."

I don't know why I did not explore other options for a journalism program. The best I can say is that the obsessive compulsive disorder had me totally fixated on Ryerson and Carleton. It is as though I was rendered completely unaware that I could look elsewhere at other schools such as Mohawk, Humber, and Western. This is an example of rigidity, being set in your thinking, that you can only go two certain schools and nowhere else. If I had been thinking logically and rationally I would have done a complete search of what journalism schools were available in Ontario.

My Rise and Fall As A Reporter

Because of my obsessive compulsive disorder, I started off on the wrong foot. First of all, I regarded this job as only a temporary job until I could get into Ryerson or Carleton University. I was a city girl starting off in a parochial small town in northern Ontario and I believe that I encountered a culture clash.

Unlike my present life in Hamilton, where I have served on the Hamilton Historical Board, in Iroquois Falls I had no interest in getting involved in the community, or any interest in local history. This lack of interest insulted Bill Cavell, Mrs. Hall, and the production staff.

I was a city girl with a university degree. Mrs. Hall also had a university degree, from the University of Lethbridge in Alberta. Bill Cavell had started in the newspaper business in his native town of Owen Sound and worked his way up to be a publisher in Iroquois Falls over many years. Neither he nor the production staff had any education beyond high school.

Looking back, I may have snubbed the newspaper production staff. Cavell told me that they had complained that I was treating them like idiots. I considered that in snitching on me, they were employing kindergarten style tactics and I ignored them.

When Cavell picked me up at the Timmins Airport, to drive me back to Iroquois Falls, he brought with him a third member of the editorial staff, Margaret Southall. Margaret told me that she did not do daily reporting. Her job was to put together a magazine which was a supplement for the weekly newspaper. Margaret was a blonde lady of around 30 years of age. Before starting on <u>The Enterprise</u> several years before, she had been a newspaper woman in a small town in England.

Cavell took me to the apartment building where I would be renting a bachelor apartment and after I dropped off my luggage, he drove me to the home of Mrs. Hall, who would be my immediate boss. As soon as I had left, Mrs. Hall encouraged me to call her Boyne, and warned me to beware of Margaret.

"Margaret is Bill Cavell's mistress," Boyne said, "They are living together in an apartment in back of <u>The Enterprise</u> offices. It is not strictly a private relationship, but carries on into the work situation."

"That's strange, I said to her, "When he came down to Toronto to interview me, he said that he had married his high school sweetheart in Owen Sound and he and his wife had five grown children."

"Let me tell you the story, "Boyne continued, "Bill and his wife, Lynne and their children were a very prominent family in Iroquois Falls. Lynn Cavell is a very nice woman."

"Anyway, several years ago he hired Margaret to put together our magazine. She was a single woman and he was married. Now, when you are single and working with another woman's husband, you should behave circumspectly. Margaret did not. She shamelessly chased Bill and he fell for her. When she had to leave the office to find material for the magazine, he drove her to where she had to go. The next thing we knew, they were together, ostensibly to work, all the time. Bill flaunted Margaret shamelessly all over town."

"Poor Lynn Cavell would come to the office to cry on my shoulder, dying inside. She knew that her marriage was over. Bill did not leave her immediately, but he took vacations with Margaret. The first year that Margaret worked here, he and Margaret travelled together to the Fiji Islands. The following year they went to Tahiti."

"When she had been here for three years, Margaret left to take an editor's job on a weekly newspaper in Oakville, near Toronto. We all thought that their relationship with Bill was over and we all breathed a sigh of relief, especially Lynn. That was two years ago. But about a month ago, Margaret returned. Now Lynn Cavell is gone and Bill and Margaret are living together."

I have to admit that after I heard this amazing story, I was horrified. Thanks to my obsessive compulsive disorder, I developed a jaundiced view of my publisher and Margaret, and they picked up on it. When Cavell complained that the production staff snitched on me, I now wonder if he was not man enough to say that the complainants were himself and Margaret. After the Christmas season was over in January, he and Margaret took a trip to Acapulco.

Looking back, my somewhat restricted view of life did not allow me to realize that relationships between bosses and employees have always existed and have been commonplace. I should not have been so surprised and angered by it and just ignored the whole thing as it was none of my business.

When Cavell fired me in February, he did not fault my reporting, but said that my personality was unsuitable for the newspaper. I asked him for a letter of reference, but he laughed in my ear. You see, he did not have the backbone to fire me in person, but he telephoned me my apartment at the end of the first week in February.

"Are you kidding?" he asked me, "I fired you and you want a letter of recommendation. Forget it."

Because of my obsessive compulsive disorder, the firing from my reporting job traumatized me. When I returned to Toronto, my mother told me, "You have three months of experience under your belt. Look for another newspaper job."

Feeling sorry for me, Boyne gave me a letter of recommendation. But she signed it as the editor of <u>The Enterprise</u>. I photocopied the letter and sent it with my resume when I applied for another newspaper job to a weekly newspaper in Peterborough. The publisher of this weekly paper, Peter Toner, telephoned me to demand who the owner of <u>The Enterprise</u> was. I had no choice but to tell him about Bill Cavell. Peter asked me, "Why didn't this Mr. Cavell give you the letter of reference?" I answered, "He wouldn't give me a reference because he fired me. Needless to say, Peter Toner just turned down my application without an interview.

I gave up getting another job as a reporter because I was afraid that no other newspaper published would take a chance on me. I applied for a writing job in the public relations department of a company, because, after all, I am a writer. When I was called for an interview, I did well, but the interviewer would not accept my letter of reference from Boyne. The interviewer insisted on calling Cavell. I never heard from her again.

At this point, Uncle Isadore, who was working as the Comptroller of Toronto Cartons in Scarborough, set up a meeting for me with Vivian Hedman, a friend of his who owned an employment agency. Vivian called up Cavell to see what he would say about me. I remember that Vivian was absolutely horrified at the nasty way in which he bad-mouthed me. I gave her photocopies of some of my news stories so that she could see that I was a good reporter. Vivian said to me, "Mr. Cavell said that you were rude and insulting to your co-workers and that, even though your reporting was satisfactory, he could not keep you on at The Enterprise."

I was crestfallen at this news. My career as a newspaper reporter was over before it had started. I was afraid to re-apply to Carleton University's School of Journalism because one of the application requirements was a letter of reference from a newspaper publisher.

Looking back on my job on The Enterprise now, three points occur to me. One is that Boyne Hall was upset with Bill Cavell. He and his family were prominent in Iroquois Falls, and them Margaret came along and ended his marriage. Boyne Hall must have been desperate to confide in somebody, otherwise she would not have told me a story about a relationship that was essentially none of my business.

Secondly, I arrived in Iroquois Falls knowing nothing of my publisher's relationship with Margaret. Cavell must have felt guilty about his relationship. Otherwise, why would he care what a total stranger from Toronto thought of it? With my uncontrolled obsessive compulsive disorder and in my youthful naivety, I must have given off vibrations to him and Margaret that they did not like.

Thirdly, I have figured out why he hired reporters for the Christmas season and fired them the following February. He did not have the money to pay for an extra reporter all year round. Cavell was taking money out of the newspaper to fund his relationship with Margaret. Probably, he was also paying alimony to his wife, Lynn. He was not man enough to admit that he had fired me because he needed what would otherwise have been my salary because he was running with his mistress to the South Pacific. He had to say that I was a lousy person.

When I told my revelations to my mother in a recent telephone conversation, my mother said bitterly, "That son-of-a-bitch in Iroquois Falls ruined your life. When you were working on Excalibur at York University you were a real dynamo. After you got that bad reference from Bill Cavell, you lost your personality and became a wimp. You gave up on being a writer and you were wrecked.

My final opportunity for a newspaper job came from Vivian Hedman. The Financial Times of Canada, located at Leslie Street and Eglinton Avenue East, was seeking a new copy typist. They had a fabulous copy typist already, but they were looking for a replacement because the newspaper was moving to new offices at 789 Yonge Street. The current typist lived in Don Mills and wanted to find another job there.

Vivian presented my qualifications to the publisher's secretary, Judy Gravelle. Judy called me in for an interview. Although she thought that I was suitable for the job, she wanted to contact Bill Cavell. After she contacted Cavell, she had second thoughts about hiring me. Vivian refused to withdraw my application and Judy had a change of mind.

"If Debbie really wants the job," Judy said to Vivian, "our typist is taking a three- week holiday. Debbie can come and work for us during these three weeks."

Uncle Isadore was pleased that I finally had another opportunity for a newspaper job. "Here is your chance to prove that Cavell is a liar," he said to me, "Just because you didn't get along with a group of hicks on a rinky-dink newspaper in a small town doesn't mean you can't work with professional people working for a Toronto newspaper."

I was thankful for the three week job. I was so eager to prove that I could get along with people that I became a wimp. At the end of the three weeks, Judy Gravelle called me into her office. "We can't hire you as a copy typist because your qualifications are more suited to a reporting or a writing job. We don't have any right now.

"Why do you say that?" I asked.

"Vivian Hedman sent us copies of your news stories which you previously had photocopied yourself and given in to her," Judy answered, "Your reporting and writing skills show us that we cannot hire you as a copy typist."

Well, folks, that was the end of my newspaper career. During my time there I wrote 28 articles and took 9 photographs.

My Rise and Fall As A Secretary

"Why on earth did you become a secretary when you returned to Toronto from Iroquois Falls?" Dr. Henry Fenigstein asked me at our initial meeting, when he accepted me into his group therapy sessions. "Why didn't you go back to York University, study to get better marks, and go for a PH.D. in Political Science?" Dr. Fenigstein, owner of the North York Psychotherapy Clinic at Bathurst Street and Glencairn Avenue, will be discussed further on in this memoir.

"Basically," I answered, "I was afraid that if I studied for a PH.D., I would never get married. None of my female professors at York University were married. Whereas girls I knew who went to work as secretaries in offices after they finished their three-year university degrees did get married."

I had no idea what to do with my life after my perceived failure as a journalist. I decided to try my hand at the advertising end of the media industry. In my mind, what was the difference between writing news stories or writing advertising copy?

Humber College offered an advertising diploma as part of its School of Business. But to be accepted into it, you had to submit an application package along with samples of advertising copy. You had to have sales experience, because advertising involved selling. Since I had neither, I could not apply to Humber College.

On the other hand, I took out of the library and read what was considered the successful business woman's Bible, <u>Having It All</u> by Helen Gurley Brown, who was once the editor-in-chief of <u>Vogue Magazine</u>. She illustrated stories of several very successful advertising account executives who had started out as secretaries. Helen said that a woman who worked out as a secretary could advance into any department of a company, including the advertising department. Thanks to my obsessive compulsive disorder symptoms and my youthful naivety, I believed her. I decided that to get into advertising, the secretarial route was the way to go.

Community colleges offered secretarial diplomas, but, when I inquired, admissions people told me that I would find their programs boring. On the other hand, Shaw College, located on Yonge Street between Lawrence and Eglinton, offered an Accelerated Business Course diploma. This program, which could be completed within nine months, offered special courses to train university graduates for jobs as administrative assistants to company presidents. Shaw College's program offered courses such as Business Organization and Management and Advanced Office Practice, in addition to basic typing and shorthand. Advanced Office Practice included researching and writing a formal report for the company president, and operating a calculating machine.

Shaw College admitted me with open arms. I was all excited about the Accelerated Business Course. Because of my obsessive compulsive disorder symptoms, I lacked the focus to research the business world properly. If I had, I would have found out that Helen Gurley Brown was actually describing a lost world. At the time I trained to be a secretary, companies no longer offered secretaries upward mobility. It was the case of once a secretary, always a secretary. For specific departments, such as advertising, department heads hired new people directly from Advertising Diploma programs and no longer picked copywriters from the secretarial pool. Also, for jobs as advertising account executives, companies required a Master's Degree in Business Administration.

All of this information I only found out after being fired from the following advertising jobs: Norwich Union Life Assurance Company, in their Advertising Department; the Royal York Hotel, in their Marketing and Catering Department; McLauchlan, Mohr, Massey Advertising; and McKim Advertising. I got these jobs through the Shaw College Placement Service.

I got the following secretarial jobs through temporary agencies: Branson Hospital; Can Labs; Fenco-Lavalin Engineering; Ministry of Labour; Ministry of Community and Social Services. I was fired from all these temporary jobs.

I saw advertisements in the <u>Toronto Star</u> for permanent jobs as a secretary. I was hired and fired from the following: A.C. MacPherson and Co. Stockbrokers; Gordon Daly Grenadier Securities; Bialik Hebrew Day School; and Canada Life Assurance Company. In addition to this one I can add Bell Canada where I was hired after I went to their office and applied. I was fired at a later time.

When I was hired at Norwich Union Life Assurance Society and at A.C. MacPherson, I was hired directly by the person who would be my immediate superior. At the other companies, I was hired by the

Personnel Officer, and did not meet my immediate superior until I started. In these situations, my immediate supervisors did not like me, and worked behind the scenes to get me fired from the start. My obsessive compulsive disorder symptoms affected my work habits and gave my supervisors ammunition against me. I talked too much, fought with everyone, and was too slow at performing my tasks.

At MacLauchlan, Mohr, Massey Advertising, I was hired by one of the partners, Allan Massey, who was related to the famous Massey family. Massey hired me to be a secretary to his wife, Michelle, who was the top account executive, and to the Comptroller.

Michelle Massey disliked me from the start. The Comptroller, Richard Ponesse, interestingly enough, liked me personally, but did not think that I was suitable for the job.

"If Allan Massey had set up a meeting for you with me, instead of hiring you himself, I would have turned you down as an employee," Ponesse said in my termination interview, "Hiring you was a mistake. You should not have been hired."

He went on to say, "Because I like you, I am going to give you a generous severance package. You will have enough money to allow you to look around for the right job, and not just grab the first job that comes along. I further recommend that you drop the idea of a career in advertising."

My first interview for a job after this firing from MacLauchlan, Mohr, Massey was at Peggy Dean and Associates which was a personnel agency. At this interview I was asked a strange question.

"Is it true that Allan Massey is an alcoholic?" the interviewer asked me. "I have heard rumors that Al Massey has a drinking problem."

"I don't know," I answered, "but come to think of it, he tended to act strangely around the company. If he drinks, that would explain his behaviour."

After that the interviewer went on to tell me that I was registered with the agency and that they would call me if a suitable job opening came up. I never heard from them. Right after that the Shaw College Placement Office sent me to McKim Advertising.

I should have listened to Ponesse, and not bother with advertising agencies anymore. But I did not listen to him, and went on to another advertising agency, McKim Advertising. I failed there because I was hired by the Personnel Director and when I started work, the chief Account Executive to whom I reported did not like me. He said that I worked too slowly and my personality was not compatible with his. So I was fired again.

As you can see I went from one secretarial job disaster to another. My obsessive compulsive disorder affected both my behaviour and my job performance. At each termination interview, my bosses found fault with my personality, not with my office skills. I did not pick up right away on their assessment that I was too slow for an office job because I had always been slow. I did not realize that being a slowpoke in an office gave my co-workers the impression that I was being deliberately lazy, and that this laziness was part of my personality.

In each termination interview my bosses said that I was too slow and that I had a "bad personality". Well, I did appear to have a personality problem. I refused to have personal conversations with my co-workers because I felt superior to them due to my university degree. When I was asked what I had studied, my answer always was, "Don't be a hyprocrite. You never went to university, yourself, so don't pretend to be interested in my studies." Because of my obsessive compulsive disorder I cried at each termination interview.

Each time a boss fired me, I could feel him or her gloating over how they had accomplished their highest calling in life by firing someone. For example, I remember my boss at Norwich Union Life Assurance Society, laughing at me when I left her office in tears. She went into another executive colleague's office and shouted at him, within my earshot, "I did it, I fired

Debbie. This is the first time I have ever fired a staff member, and it felt terrific. She may have a B.A., and I don't have a B.A., but I still have a job and she doesn't have one."

So as you can see, I was too slow for office work. My continual checking and repetitive behaviour made my work even slower. I was also unable to hold down a job because of inappropriate behaviour and my personality and was continually being fired. My inappropriate behaviour consisted of giggling and ineptitude at complicated tasks and constant verbal repetition and making inappropriate statements. I felt that I was superior to my co-workers because I had a university degree and refused to have personal conversations with them. I apparently could not function properly in a work environment.

I kept looking for secretarial jobs hoping that the next one would be successful. But none of them worked out. I thought that I was a bad person because I had been fired from all of my secretarial jobs. When I finally went back to York University's Atkinson College to finish my Honours Bachelor of Arts in Political Science Degree and then the Master of Library Science Degree program at the University of Toronto, I was afraid to tell classmates and professors that I had been fired from secretarial jobs.

I now know that a person who does not have obsessive compulsive disorder will realize that they are not suited to office work after they lose a few jobs.

They will just go back to university or community college and educate themselves for another type of work. They are also not ashamed of having been fired.

Also, I also know that, when I found that I enjoyed reporting for <u>Excalibur</u> rather than studying political science, I should have transferred from York University to the four-year Journalism Program at Carleton University. I could probably have gotten in as a transfer student. Since at Carleton I would actually have learned how to write for the mass media, I would probably have gotten better marks and not lost my writing ability.

My Fourth Year at Atkinson College, York University

It was Dr. Henry Fenigstein, owner of the North York Psychotherapy Clinic, who told me to go back to university to complete my fourth year. Dr. Fenigstein will be discussed later in this memoir.

First of all, I want to say that I did not want to go back to Atkinson College to study. Before I began at Atkinson College, I applied with my mediocre marks from my three year B.A. degree to the graduate level M.L.S. degree at the Faculty of Library Science at the University of Toronto. The Faculty Registrar, Dr. Alvin Bregman, sent me a rejection letter in which he asked me to return to a university to complete a fourth year of study, and invited me to re-apply to the program with presumably better marks.

I had gone to York University for three years knowing nothing about University of Toronto. But in the intervening years, I had met graduates of the University of Toronto and had learned that the University of Toronto was a prestigious university.

I could not afford financially to study full-time because of my father's untimely death from diabetes.

I decided to apply to the University of Toronto's part-time Woodsworth College, as a transfer student. Their Admissions Office rejected me, saying that, they felt that I had been away from university for a number of years, so I was no longer in an "academic frame of mind". Ever so reluctantly, I applied to Atkinson College at York University. I received an acceptance letter from a lady named Suzin Ferris in the Admissions Office. Suzin said that, in order to receive an Honours B.A. in Political Science, I had to complete two political theory courses, one at third year level and one at fourth year level, one of two third year courses, either Canadian government and Politics or Political Economy of Canada, and two other fourth year courses of my choice.

My first course, completed during the Fall/Winter Term, was Government and Politics of Ontario with the late Donald C. MacDonald, a former leader of the Ontario New Democratic Party. It was thoroughly enjoyable.

My fun began when I started off the Summer Term with Canadian Government and Politics, taught by Hector Massey. Dr. Massey was teaching his first course after obtaining his PH.D. from York University and he was totally disorganized. He did not present the class with either a course outline nor course requirements at the first class. We were all surprised. But we all figured that he would get his act together in time for the second class.

Well, we arrived for the second class to find that he had cancelled it and the two succeeding classes due to "important work" that he was doing for one of the political parties and also because a family member had died. Everybody in the class was stupefied. We did not want to fail the course. Because of my obsessive compulsive disorder, I panicked, thinking that I would have a failure on my new record. I ran to the main office at Atkinson College and dropped the course. The clerk who served me said, "We have passed the allotted time for you to drop this course, so we can only give you a partial refund."

When I got home, my mother was furious. "You should have waited to see what the rest of the class was doing before you lost money on a course, "she yelled at me. "If the jerk is going to spend the whole summer messing around with a political party and running to funerals, he still has to give you credit for the course."

"But we lost three classes, I protested. "So far, we haven't had any lectures or been given assignments. How can we have the course?"

"That is his problem," my mother answered. "How dare you just quit a course without a full refund!"

After her tantrum, I was cringing. Because of my obsessive compulsive disorder, I was afraid of her anger. The next morning, I telephoned the Atkinson College Chairperson of Political Science, Dr. David Davies.

"I want to lodge a complaint against Dr. Hector Massey," I said. "I also want to get a full refund from the course. The clerk in the Main Office told me that I am not entitled to a full refund."

"Let me talk to Dr. Massey and find out what happened," he answered, "before we do anything."

A half hour later, I received a telephone call from Dr. Massey.

""I belong to the Ontario Progressive Conservative Party," he said, "and we are preparing for a fall election. I thought that I could make the class better after I finish this work. We are studying government and politics, after all. I was only planning on cancelling one class. Then my brother was killed in a car accident, and it gave me such a shock that I couldn't function."

"You have cancelled three classes," I answered. "How do you plan to make them up. As far as I am concerned, the course is a complete disaster."

"As far as I am concerned, you are a heartless person," he yelled, and hung up.

Whereupon, I telephoned Dr. Davies and yelled at him, "Dr. Massey is a nut and I demand a dull refund. I am losing an entire term because of this crap."

"I can see that you are very upset," Dr. Davies said, "and I will write a letter to the Main Office instructing them to give you a full refund immediately," he promised.

That afternoon, a clerk from the Atkinson College Central Administrative Office telephoned me. She said, "We have received an internal communication from Dr. Davies requesting us to give you a full refund for Canadian Government and Politics. It will take us two weeks to process the refund, and, after that we will mail it to you."

So I wasted the whole summer. The course was offered again in the Fall/Winter Term. When I found out that Hector Massey would be teaching it again I was furious.

'Do you mean to say that, in all of Atkinson College, indeed, all of York University, you cannot find another professor to teach it?" I demanded.

Instead of answering me, the clerk who took my payment changed the subject. "We can sign you up for Political Economy of Canada, with Professor Daniel Drache," she said, placating me.

When I first glanced at the course outline for Political Economy of Canada, the course seemed extremely interesting and Professor Drache seemed to be organized. He sent the class to the university bookstore to purchase the required textbooks and he sold us a package of individual readings. The course outline contained lecture topics and the course requirements.

His first two lectures went well. Then a new problem developed. The office staff of York University went on strike. Professor Drache telephoned the class to tell us that classes were cancelled until the strike was over. Picket lines had been set up at the entrances to the university and he was not crossing them.

"Why aren't you crossing the picket lines?" I asked him, "What do you care about the office staff?"

"The secretaries are the arms and legs of the university," he answered. "We faculty members couldn't get along without them. If we faculty members cancel classes, it will bring pressure to bear on the university administrators and they will give the secretaries what they want."

"I have paid for a course," I protested, "I don't think it is fair of you to cancel classes." Because of my obsessive compulsive disorder symptoms, I yelled at him, "You are a jerk. You are just like Hector Massey."

"Don't you dare compare me to Hector Massey." he answered angrily, "That idiot has never taught any courses before now. Whereas I have been teaching for years and I know what I am doing. I will call you when the strike ends and classes resume." With that, he hung up.

Well, after that, I was on the wrong foot with Professor Drache. It turned out that most of the class was mad at him for cancelling classes that we had paid for. When the strike was over two weeks later, he inserted into the course two Saturday lectures as make-up classes. But only a few students, including myself, were able to attend the Saturday classes because the majority of the class had prior commitments. In addition to that, the course material contained very technical economic concepts and very little actual political content. Most of the students, including myself, got a mediocre mark in the course. I got a C Plus, which was a pass for Honours students, and C Plus was the class average.

During the Summer Term, I completed the required third year political theory course, taught by Professor Michael Michi. He was actually a PH.D. student of history and he had been a high school history teacher. I got a very good mark in the course, although I found that the abstract political theory exacerbated my obsessive compulsive disorder symptoms by making the theory difficult to grasp. I felt like I was being overwhelmed with too much abstract and confusing information that seemed useless and meaningless to me.

When the next Fall/Winter Term arrived a fourth year course opened up, Canadian Prime Ministers, taught by Hector Massey. The Atkinson College Political Science Department Secretary, Louise Jacobs, told me that I was not welcome in Hector Massey's course. The other fourth year courses were in Political Economy and Public Administration. Louise recommended that because of my mediocre performance in Political Economy of Canada, I not take these courses.

"I can offer you an alternative," Louise suggested. "Would you like to do a Directed Reading with Donald C. MacDonald? I will check with him to see if he will take you on for a Directed Reading."

Later on the same day Donald C. MacDonald telephoned me to say, "I will be delighted to oversee you on a Directed Reading course, but I have no idea how to complete the paperwork. You will have to do the paperwork with Louise Jacobs."

Well, I completed a very successful reading course on The Government Party a book by Reginald Whitaker. From there, I proceeded to my final course during the following Summer Term, a fourth year course called The Demise of Communism: Alternative Political Theories taught by Dr. Max Nemni. Dr. Nemni was a Political Theory Professor at Laval University, who had received his Ph.D in Political Science from York University. He was at York's Atkinson College teaching for the Summer Term.

This was a seminar course and not a lecture course and I was unable to grasp the political theories. Having to do seminars on theories that I did not understand threw me into a rage.

Dr. Nemni, began the course by saying, "My goal in this course is to find out what you think, in your own words, of the political theories that we will be discussing."

My inability to grasp the theory without lectures left me very frustrated. I actually shouted at Dr. Nemni, "This is my final course before I graduate and I am going on to graduate school at the University of

Toronto. I am not interested in discussing anything. I just want to pass the course and move on."

To which Dr. Nemni replied, "Thinking out political theory is necessary to understand how political systems operate. If you just want to read books and take lecture notes, you are not only an automaton, but you are also childish."

While I was studying at Atkinson College, I attended a lecture series at the University of Toronto's Convocation Hall. This series featured distinguished international political science academics including John Kenneth Galbraith, Gwynne Dwyer, Robert Reich, and Tom Wolfe. Of interest to this memoir is Tom Wolfe.

Dr. Wolfe began his lecture by saying, "We live in a society in which Mom and Dad, Junior and Sis, and Spot the dog no longer matter. Middle-aged men are tossing aside long-standing, faithful wives who have borne and raised their children in favour of some loosely-moraled "Cookie" some twenty years younger than they are. These men give as their excuse that the wife no longer wants to have sex and at their age they are full of beans. Well, I think that those men are bad people who need to satisfy what is essentially a primitive urge."

After he was finished, a female student went up to the microphone and asked Dr. Wolfe, "Professor, what do you think of Freud?" He answered, "Sigmund Freud exposed the pig tracks in men's souls."

At about this time my brain was exploding uncontrollably. I was enraged because of my obsessive compulsive disorder, at what he had said. I stepped up to the microphone and shouted at him, "Dr. Wolfe, maybe you are a famous political scientist, but you are disgusting."

He in turn asked me, "Are you married or single?"

I answered, "I am single." In reply, he asked me again, "Are you sexually active?" When I answered, "None of your business," he said, "Then you are the one who is disgusting, not me."

After the lecture a few girls came up to me and congratulated me for having the guts to say what they were thinking. One of these girls said, "Don't pay him any attention. Dr. Wolfe just sounds like a typical southern United States evangelical preacher."

As I look back on this episode, I believe that I just might have laughed at Dr. Wolfe if my obsessive compulsive disorder had been under control.

University of Toronto Library School

During the period that I graduated from Atkinson College, applied to Library School at the University of Toronto, and attended and graduated from Library School was a two year period in which I was still in therapy with Dr. Fenigstein and taking Clomipramine and attending the Obsessive Compulsive Disorder Support Group. I was better but still not fully under control.

I successfully completed my final political science course at Atkinson College and received my honours B.A. at the Autumn Convocation. I had reapplied to Library School when I was taking my final course. A week after that Dr. Bregman at the Faculty of Library Science telephoned me.

"Your final year at York University has given us a far superior scenario of your ability to do academic work at the graduate level, Debbie, "he said, "We are going to send a memo to the School of Graduate Studies asking that you be admitted to our faculty."

I was very dizzy with excitement. I was finally going to be a student at the University of Toronto, one of Canada's most prestigious universities. Because of my obsessive compulsive disorder, I could not focus on the actual career that I was to be educated for. If I had done so, I would have applied to different libraries, saying that I had been admitted to library school, and that I was looking for a part-time job. I would also have visited the faculty office to take a look at course outlines and requirements. Instead, the glittering lights of the university beckoned me and until January of the following year, when I would start my studies, I spent my time exploring the St. George campus.

The faculty had a cocktail party during my first week there to welcome new students. At this party, I met my new classmates. Many of them were foreign students from all over the world. There were also Canadians with PH.D.'s in academic disciplines. Still others were second and third generation University of Toronto students who had done all of their undergraduate work at the university.

Although the foreign students and the PH.D. graduates welcomed me, the graduates of the University of Toronto laughed at me when I told them that I had a degree from York University.

One of the elite students, who came from a very prominent Toronto family, said to me, "York is a joke as far as universities are concerned. They give a degree to anybody. You will bomb out here if you are not careful. To see what I mean, go over there and talk to Jennifer Osther. She also went to York."

To stick up for myself, I answered, "My Uncle Stanley got a Master's Degree in Business Administration from York, and he works for the Ministry of the Treasury and Intergovernmental Affairs."

"Oh, the M.B.A. curriculum is not specific to York. It is a standard curriculum for all universities. Just like our library courses are standard worldwide librarian courses. We are accredited by the American Library Association. Whereas, York makes up rinky-dink courses." was his response.

After that, I developed an inferiority complex. I found myself trying to ingratiate myself with my classmates, instead of focussing on my studies and looking for a part-time library job. This happened because of my obsessive compulsive disorder. I became obsessed with everyone liking me to the point where I chased after them and, reflecting back, I probably made a fool out of myself. I made friends with two students, Sharon Moynes and Linda Morse, but that was all. I also tried to ingratiate myself with my professors. The results were that they thought that I acted strange and developed a wrong impression of me.

After completing one course per semester at Atkinson College, I found taking four courses per semester for four semesters overwhelming. The amount of time required to attend classes, do the reading, and complete assignments was enormous. If my obsessive compulsive disorder had made me a slowpoke at York University, I was doubly a slowpoke at the University of Toronto. I was worried that, if I worked part-time, I would not pass the courses.

The Faculty of Library Science had its own library with readings and reference materials. Unlike York University, where the professors had sold us packages of readings, we had to read the required readings individually in our library. This was also the beginning of computer laboratories in universities. Instead of typing assignments, the assignments had to be keyed into word processing software on the computers supplied by the faculty in our computer lab.

I was unable to multi-task, so I worked on my assignments one by one in priority sequence. If I finished an assignment I had to enter it on the computer right away. If I could not get a computer right away because they were all taken, I got angry at the other students who were using the computers.

Academic writing at the University of Toronto was stiff and formal, leaving no room for individual creativity.

Since I commuted to the university from my home at Don Mills and McNicoll, I found the hour long commute from home to the university exacerbated my obsessive compulsive disorder. My mother supported me financially, but reluctantly, while I was studying, but she kept urging me to get a part-time job in a library. The faculty encouraged students to work while they were studying as a prelude to getting permanent full-time jobs.

The Library Science program was fully available on a part-time basis, but had to be completed within six years. In addition the pass was a B. Some of the students had been A students as undergraduates but many had not been, so they found it difficult to keep up their grades.

Every assignment for every course was crucial in completing the degree, so we could not afford to blow any assignments. Jennifer Osther complained to me about this, "I like a course in which the professor gives one assignment to start with that is only worth a small percentage. That way you get to see what the professor is looking for and how they mark. My professors at York were like that. Here, if you get a mediocre mark on an assignment, you are finished."

All of the students who worked full-time had to cut back their course load from four per semester to two or three. Some of the students cut back to part-time study even though they were not working part-time.

One fellow whom I met in the computer lab said to me, "The time required to complete all of the assignments is horrendous. You have to literally live here if you study full-time. Either that, or you have to buy your own computer and not be dependent on the computer lab here."

Looking back, I see that I should have lived in residence rather than commuting and I should have worked part-time. The students who lived in residence helped each other to complete assignments and students who worked part-time in a library were able to get help from their co-workers.

During my third semester, I took a course called Historical Manuscript and Archival Collections with a professor whose name I cannot recall. In this course, we learned the history of objects that are used every day in libraries, archives, and business offices. We also learned how to catalogue exhibits on display in archives.

At the fourth class, the professor gave us an enormous brown envelope containing pictures and writing samples to be catalogued. This brown envelope was awkward and bulky to carry. It also cluttered up my bedroom at home.

Within a week, I had finished cataloguing everything. I wanted to bring this package to the following class and give it back to the professor. Then I remembered that the fifth class was going to be a tour of the Archives of Ontario. Fed up with the bulky, clumsy envelop, I took it to the Archives of Ontario anyway.

When the professor saw the envelope, she asked me, "Would you save it and bring it to the next class, please? It is awkward for me to carry it around here."

I answered, "This big envelope is cumbersome. I don't want it anymore. Either you take it, professor, or it goes into the garbage."

My sharp answer stunned the professor. She silently took the envelope.

During my fourth and final semester, I almost failed a reference course taught by Professor Claire England. I started off on the wrong foot with her by saying, "The comprehensive reference guide that you have given us is so disorganized that I can't find anything in it."

"That is not a tactful thing to say." she answered. It turned out that she had compiled this reference guide.

She retaliated when she did our first assignment, in which we rated the readership level of different magazines. One of these was <u>The New Yorker</u>. About <u>The New Yorker</u>, I wrote the following assessment, "The trademark of <u>The New Yorker</u> is a long-haired gentleman in a top hat and wearing a frock coat writing on a desk putting a quill to the paper. Not for the unlettered masses is <u>The New Yorker</u>. It is meant to appeal to the upper classes."

When she gave the class back our assignments, she did not give mine back, but asked me to make an appointment to see her in her office. When I met with her, she said, "I regret to inform you that you have failed this assignment."

"Why?" I asked.

"Because the way that you write is not an appropriate style for academic writing. For example, you should have rated <u>The New Yorker</u> with a sentence like, I rate <u>The New Yorker</u> to be suitable for, etc. I wish I could pass this assignment but I can't. I will allow you to re-write this assignment if you will do it properly."

"My other professors have not faulted my writing style," I protested, "Why do you?"

"It isn't your writing style, "she answered, "It is your whole attitude. You are a pretentious person. At this university you cannot write the same way that you can write fiction. You have to write sentences like, "The cat jumped on the table." We are very conservative here and you are writing like a pretentious snob."

To save my performance in the course, I did complete a make-up assignment and felt like a pupil in kindergarten while I did it. But this took time away from my other courses. Afraid of failing the reference course, I made an appointment with Dean Adele Fasick.

Dean Fasick said to me, "Don't worry about failing. You are an adult in a Master's Degree program at a university, not a child in school. If you fail a course, we give you the option to have your assignment re-evaluated by another faculty member before we put a failure on your record."

By catering to Dr. England's conservative whims, I ended up passing the course. Looking back, I think that she passed me because she was afraid of looking like a fool if another faculty member passed me after she had failed me. I also think that instead of rewriting a perfectly well-written assignment to please her, I should have dropped the course and taken it the following semester with another professor. When she failed me I panicked.

Looking back, I should have bought my own computer. Then I would have been able to work on my assignments whenever I wanted to. I would then have been able to get a part-time library job and working while I was taking my courses. I, however, did not know anything about computers and what to buy and I had no one to help me.

A Bad Obsessive Compulsive Disorder Episode at Library School

In my fourth semester I took a course entitled Contemporary Publishing. It was taught by Ian Montagnes, an adjunct professor, who was the publisher of the University of Toronto Press. My highest mark A+ was obtained in this course. I guess that I would also say that this was my favourite course, because as a wannabe writer, I felt at home in it.

In Contemporary Publishing, our major assignment was to form groups of four people. Each group had to become a publishing company and publish one small book. This small book was to be presented to the final class by all of the groups. Either the whole group could present the book, or the group could pick one person as its representative. We had one required reading, a reference book which would show us the template for the publishing company.

My group consisted of myself, Walter Eisenbeis, Grace Griffiths, and Sherrill Robinson. We met once or twice per week in the Library School lounge to work on the book.

Both Walter and Grace were able to spend more time on this assignment than me because they both had Apple laptop computers. Walter lived in residence and could work on his computer whenever he wanted. Grace was selected to read the book for all of us. She was able to read and work on her computer, while she was travelling from her home in Etobicoke to the university. Sherrill had a teenaged daughter to look after, and she could not afford her own computer, so she was not able to contribute much to the group either.

Grace said to me, two weeks after the class began, "Debbie you should buy your own laptop computer. That way you could work on this course, for that matter, all of your courses, while you are commuting from your home to the university and back."

"I can't work while I am commuting," I answered. "The noise on the bus and the subway puts me to sleep." What I told her was a white lie. I could not focus on my work during the commute because of my obsessive compulsive disorder.

The four of us ended up creating a publishing company called Four Winds Press, and we produced a book called <u>The Four Winds of Learning</u>. The book was about our undergraduate education. Grace talked about her education in Australia. Walter talked about his education in India. I talked about studying at York University and reporting for <u>Excalibur</u>, and Sherrill talked about her education in the West Indies. Grace and Walter produced the entire book on their Apple computers. Because the library school computer lab had a different operating system, Sherrill and I had to let Grace and Walter type everything. Grace and Walter went together to a print shop to run off five copies of our book for distribution to the rest of the class.

When we had our last meeting before the final class, I said to Walter and Grace, "I am sorry that I could not help more with putting out the book. I have obsessive compulsive disorder."

"Do you really?" Walter asked. When I answered, "yes," he went on, "My brother has obsessive compulsive disorder and so does my sister. Not to worry. Grace and I will handle the presentation.

Four Winds Press procured for us an A+, the highest mark in the class. Because Grace and Walter had done more work than me, I felt guilty about the mark. I became afraid that Walter and Grace would go to Ian Montagnes and complain about my less than stellar performance.

I telephoned Grace twice to ask if she was going to complain about me. The first time she answered, "No, Debbie. Don't worry. Sherrill did not contribute that much either, because she has a daughter." The second time she answered, "Debbie, I was a little miffed at first, but you told us about your disability. Besides, tattling to the teacher on fellow students is a kindergarten style tactic. We are adults in graduate school."

Even after Grace reassured me twice, I was worried that Walter would complain about me to Professor Montagnes. I telephoned Walter twice as well. The first time he answered, "No, I have not complained to the professor and I will not. Forget about it." The second time, he answered, "I already told you that I didn't. Debbie, please get a grip on yourself and go for help to your psychiatrist."

I was still worried that Grace or Walter would snitch on me, so I made an appointment to see Dean Adele Fasick. Dean Fasick said, "Debbie, I don't know what has happened in your life to make you so worried. But rest assured that we have never in this faculty had a situation in which students have tattled to a professor against their classmates. Even if they did, the professor would call you in and ask for your version of the story. We are a Graduate Studies Faculty in a university, not a kindergarten."

Needless to say, I am not proud of this episode in my life.

Obsessive Compulsive Disorder Confessions at Library School

It was while I was in my fourth semester that my friend, Sharon Moynes, advised me to tell my professors and classmates that I had obsessive compulsive disorder. I had previously told her because I was very slow at completing my academic work and my exhibiting strange behaviour such as repeating a lot and asking for reassurance a lot. I followed her advice and told everybody. Back then, nobody had ever heard of it. Professor Patricia Fleming, who taught Analytical and Historical Bibliography and Research Collections in Canadiana, asked me to describe it for her.

Dr. Fleming asked me, "Exactly how does this disorder of yours affect me?"

I answered, "I am very slow and completing assignments and I am afraid to take a part-time job because if I do I might not complete the course requirements."

She answered, "Well, I don't know what to say."

My Cataloguing courses Professor, Lynn Howarth, was the only one who even knew what obsessive compulsive disorder is. I remember her saying, "Deborah, with all of your daily struggle against your disability, I am surprised that you have the stamina to, not just complete university, but to complete a Master's Degree as well. I admire you very much and I think that you have much to pat yourself on the back for."

None of my other professors and none of my classmates made any comments to me about my obsessive compulsive disorder.

Looking back, I wonder if I should have followed Sharon's advice. Words coming out of a professor's mouth are cheap and cost the professor nothing. It is their actual behaviour afterwards that counts.

An applicant for a library job in the Toronto Public Library System has to supply three references. Because of my failed secretarial jobs, I had no employer references, and I had to rely on my professors. For all of her encouraging words when I asked Dr. Howarth for a reference, she answered, "Deborah, I must graciously decline. I only know you as a student, not as an employee."

When I approached Dr. Fleming for a reference, she answered, "Debbie, I worked in the Toronto Public Library system before I got my PH.D. They won't accept academic references unless you are a high school student applying for a part-time job as a page. With an M.L.S. graduate, they presume that you have worked part-time and summers while you are studying, and they want employer references. When you are at work, you behave differently than when you are studying, and I have not had a chance to observe you in a work situation."

"So what should I do?" I asked her.

"Get yourself a job in a private library just to get work experience and to get an employer reference," Dr. Fleming answered.

Incidentally, I tried applying for a job in the University of Toronto Library system. I found out that to work as a librarian in a university library, at any university, I would have to go back to York or any other university and complete a Master's Degree in Political Science. Since I could not face doing that, I would not be able to apply for a library job at a university. So I was restricted to finding a job in a private library.

The entire situation about applying for library jobs is ridiculous. A person cannot get work experience in a library if they cannot get a library job. If a person has received his graduate degree in library science then academic reference should be accepted if they have no library work experience. A person should not need a master's degree in a specific subject discipline to work in an academic library. Their honour's degree should be acceptable credentials along with the master's degree in library science. They should not be restricted by what their undergraduate major was and whether they have a further master's degree in the same subject. The whole purpose of the Master's Degree in Library Science is to graduate someone who is well-rounded in the subject and is capable of working in any type of library. Yet the reality is different and preposterous.

Seeing Social Workers

Eventually, after losing a series of office jobs, I finally decided to go for psychiatric help to straighten out my life and find out what was wrong with my personality. My inability to hold down a job had triggered in me another obsessive compulsive disorder symptom, extreme anxiety. All of the psychiatrists who took OHIP were fully booked up. I was forced to see a social worker instead. I actually saw two social workers. The first one, Helen Sugar, told me to "Stop your inappropriate behaviours and everything will be fine." She telephoned Shaw College's placement officer to ask her opinion of me and why I was unable to hold down a job. The placement officer said that I was rude to her. Helen said, "Debbie is now under my tutelage and will no longer be rude to you." I was not even aware that I was rude to the placement officer.

But I was unable to change, so social worker number one, Helen Sugar, switched me to social worker number two, Heather MacPherson, to find out why I was unable to change. Heather MacPherson specialized in psychotherapy.

Heather gave me the following assessment, "Your problems are a lack of social skills and a chronic inability to get along with people", she said, "You are also either unwilling or unable to do a reasonable job in an office. Your extreme anxiety of making mistakes slows down your performance." I should mention here that my extreme anxiety was fear of making mistakes. All of my bosses had taken me to task for making mistakes. She said further, "Your parents' continual fighting is exacerbating your problems. Your mother's constant criticism is also affecting your behaviour." Heather told me to leave home. When I said that I was stuck at home because of joblessness, she said that I should move into a room in a boarding house if necessary. If I did that, I would qualify for welfare. But I was unable to change my behaviour because of the obsessive compulsive disorder and we were both frustrated. Heather, was, however, unable to make a diagnosis because she was not a doctor and also because obsessive compulsive disorder was not well known at that time.

My First Meeting With Dr. Fenigstein

After my father died, my mother joined a widows' support group at the Baycrest Centre on Bathurst Street at Wilson Avenue. In this group, she met Bunny Rosenbaum who was also a widow. Bunny had a friend, Dr. William Bell, who was a family doctor. I switched from my doctor at the time, Irving Zelcer, to Dr. Bell. I had tried to get a referral to a psychiatrist from Dr. Zelcer, but he insisted that all of the psychiatrists he knew were booked up.

I told Dr. Bell my whole life history up to that point. I told him that I was going nowhere with my therapy and was desperate to see a psychiatrist. Dr. Bell referred me to a psychiatrist at Yonge Street and Davisville Avenue, Dr. Brody. Dr. Brody told me that I needed to find out why I was unable to make friends and get along with people and hold down jobs. Dr. Brody, said that I seemed not to get along with other people because I was afraid of people and had extreme anxiety and that this was also affecting my ability to do work properly and hold down a job. He said that I needed to be in group therapy and he referred me to a psychiatrist, Dr. Henry Fenigstein, at the North York Psychotherapy Clinic at Bathurst Street and Glencairn Avenue, who ran group therapy sessions, each of which was run by a social worker. Dr. Fenigstein accepted me into these sessions at my first appointment.

After my father's untimely death, I was unable to grieve, because I had to be strong for my mother. Her sudden widowhood came as a complete shock and threw her into a depression for a few years. I remember how I had to be the tower of strength on whom she could depend. There was no time to attend to my own needs and emotions.

At my first appointment with Dr. Fenigstein, he made me fill out a questionnaire and a family history chart. The questionnaire was designed to help you decide what you wanted out of group therapy. The family history chart was designed to give him your background.

In the questionnaire, I said that I was in a rut, going nowhere in a hurry, and I wanted to straighten out my life and develop a better personality so that I would be able to get along with people.

In the family history chart, my first family member was my dead father. I laid out the whole story of his death and my mother's depression. Well, the first action that Dr. Fenigstein ever made towards me was to hug me and make me cry. I cried for an hour, half of the slotted appointment time, which was for two hours.

After I had dried my tears, Dr. Fenigstein said, "You have endured the fire and have been cleansed. Expressing your feelings like this will be so necessary in my groups. You are a strong woman and I accept you into my groups. A person who cannot weep is not strong enough for my groups because they are too weak."

My Breakthrough

When I first started the group therapy sessions, I was totally out of control. I was very rude and I asked people inappropriate questions, e.g. about their sex lives and I giggled when I thought that other people's problems were insignificant compared to mine. The other people in the group called me a b****. I did not understand why my behaviour was so bad.

At the group therapy sessions I met Elaine who had symptoms very similar to mine. Elaine was considered to be strange by everyone in the group. She could not sit still and was constantly walking back and forth. I was, however, able to sit still. Elaine could not hold down a job because she was too slow and also had problems communicating with people. She also did repetition and checking. She also had been recommended by her doctor to Dr. Fenigstein for her problems. She was on medication for what she called obsessive compulsive disorder.

I saw how Elaine was in the group and made a momentous discovery. "I have obsessive compulsive disorder." I told the group. I was told by the group leader, a social worker, who worked for Dr. Fenigstein, "Debbie, if you think you have obsessive compulsive disorder, make a private appointment to see Dr. Fenigstein. You don't have to suffer. You can take medication for obsessive compulsive disorder." The social worker told me that "Obsessive compulsive disorder is a condition in which the sufferer is missing serotonin in the brain. Serotonin is a vital component of rational thought. Without it you indulge in checking, repetitive and inappropriate behaviour, and you are very anxious."

As the therapy progressed and I began to get more under control, I developed interpersonal skills by engaging in psycho-drama with others in the group, mostly with Elaine. This allowed me to gain a better understanding of why I was behaving so badly towards others and to gain more consideration of other people's problems. The others in the group thought that it was a pleasure to be with me.

Advice From Dr. Skain

One of my worst obsessive compulsive disorder episodes happened in Toronto after I diagnosed myself thanks to Elaine, but before I got a private appointment with Dr. Fenigstein. I was visiting for the first time a gynecologist, Dr. Skain, whose office was at Keele Street and Eglinton Avenue. A routine gynecological examination plus a discussion about having children, were the reasons for this visit.

When I entered Dr. Skain's office, his secretary, Mrs. Sutherland, was on the telephone. She did not immediately notice that I was there. While still on the telephone, Mrs. Sutherland finally noticed me, but did not get off the phone.

Meanwhile, the waiting room was not that full and the doctor himself was on a steady schedule of calling patients in and letting go when they were finished. Because Mrs. Sutherland had not finished her telephone conversation and had not yet signed me in for my appointment, I began panicking that I would not be able to see Dr. Skain.

Panic was raging inside me to the point where I could not control it. The next time Dr. Skain came out to get a patient, I started screaming, "Dr. Skain, I want to lodge a complaint against Mrs. Sutherland. It is almost my turn and she is too busy talking on the telephone to acknowledge my existence."

By this time, Mrs. Sutherland was off the telephone and she did sign me in, with my OHIP number. When Dr. Skain called me in, he did not proceed directly to an examination room. Instead, he sat me down in his office, and gently asked me why I threw a tantrum. "Do you have any problems that are not gynecological?"

I answered, "Dr. Skain, I am in group therapy with Dr. Henry Fenigstein. From observing a girl named Elaine in the group I realized that I have obsessive compulsive disorder. I have to make a private appointment to see Dr. Fenigstein about getting on medication."

Dr. Skain answered, "From your little scene in the waiting room, I would say that you definitely have obsessive compulsive disorder."

"What is obsessive compulsive disorder?" I asked him.

"Obsessive compulsive disorder means that you are missing in your brain a chemical called serotonin", Dr. Skain answered.

I next said to him, "I always got high marks in school and I am completing my fourth year of study at York University's Atkinson College. In the group they tell me that I am very intelligent. I always thought that if something is missing from a person's brain, that person is retarded."

"On the contrary", Dr. Skain answered, "I would think that you are very clever, indeed. Obsessive compulsive disorder does not mean that you are retarded. As a matter of fact, geniuses have it. People with your condition are driven to accomplish great feats. For example, Napoleon Bonaparte and Julius Caesar had obsessive compulsive disorder."

After that he told me what I had already been told in the group, "You don't have to suffer. Go and get on medication."

I never did find out how Dr. Skain knew so much about obsessive compulsive disorder when most people had never even heard of it. But because I had always been a slowpoke, I had thought obsessive compulsive disorder had rendered me retarded even though in therapy sessions with the social workers, I had been told I was very intelligent. Thanks to Dr. Skain, I started even before taking the Clomipramine, feeling better about myself. Incidentally, Dr. Skain found my reproductive organs healthy but advised me not to have children because the obsessive compulsive disorder is hereditary.

Intensive Therapy With Dr. Fenigstein

In these group therapy sessions I was told that despite my drawbacks I was a very intelligent person with enormous intellectual prowess and that I was not suited for office work. They suggested that I return to university to complete my fourth year of political science and that I go on from there to graduate school. But my studying abilities were frustrated because I was still very slow at reading and writing. Other people in the group, some of whom had university degrees, also exhibited similar behaviours to myself including inability to hold down a job, feeling like a mess, giggling, inappropriate statements, keeping lists, repetition, checking, etc. These were all symptoms of obsessive compulsive disorder.

I made a private appointment and saw Dr. Fenigstein who told me that he was going to put me on two 50mg pills of Clomipramine per day. The medication, however, would not be enough to cure me. "To control your obsessive compulsive behaviour you have to work through group therapy." I needed to work through the group therapy sessions in order to get better.

Looking back, after I took the medication for the first time I say to myself, "In that moment everything changed. It was the moment after I took my first dose of obsessive compulsive disorder medication. Immediately I felt like a new person and I knew everything would be all right."

From the time that I discovered that I had obsessive compulsive disorder, I took a different approach to my therapy. The neglected child could finally become an adult. I was able to nurture that child by holding a pillow in my lap. I was able to project my feelings of neglect onto the pillow. Dr. Fenigstein approved of this.

Dr. Fenigstein said that, "A person who can turn a pillow into a neglected child and nurture the pillow as if it is a child is very creative and brilliant. You are creative, Debbie, and you have repressed you creativity. A creative person is unable to do any routine job. You need to use your imagination to make money either by writing or some other creative pursuit. I suggest that you go back to university and complete your fourth year of political science."

As soon as I was on Clomipramine, Dr. Fenigstein advised me to read popular psychology books and write essays on each of them. The books included <u>The Art of Loving</u> by Erich Fromm, <u>Cutting Loose From Your Parents</u> by Ron Caplan, and <u>Man</u>

<u>The Manipulator</u> by Everett Shostrom. These books were intended to help me become an independent person and not be dependent on my mother's approval. They were to also help me to get my brain to function rationally.

"Your creative mind and your intellectual brilliance are the greatest assets you have. Use your intellect to solve your problems by reading the books and doing the scholastic exercises. Use your writing ability to say what you think of the books." was what Dr. Fenigstein told me.

<u>Reading Sigmund Freud and My Dreams</u>

Along with the books recommended by Dr. Fenigstein, I also during my therapy sessions read books of my own choosing. I picked <u>The Freud Reader</u> which was a compilation of the writings of Sigmund Freud and <u>The Interpretation of Dreams</u> by Sigmund Freud.

Sigmund Freud was the father of modern psychiatry, making his debut in the late 1800's. When I showed my mother the two books she cautioned me, "Freud is passe. Couldn't you find theories with a psychiatrist who is more modern?"

"Well, mother," I answered, "Freud was not only the father of modern psychiatry, he was also the first practitioner of psychotherapy. His theories form the roots of the psychiatric profession. I am sure that even more modern psychiatrists know that they stand on his shoulders."

When reading <u>The Freud Reader</u>, I found that I shared common traumas with Freud's patients. Just as my life had been scarred by my parents' fighting, Freud's patients had been traumatized by watching their parents have sexual intercourse. Their revelations to Freud were almost exactly the revelations that I presented in group therapy sessions.

When reading <u>The Interpretation of Dreams</u>, I learned that dreams are the keys that unlock the otherwise untouchable contents of our unconscious mind. Not only Freud's patients, but the patients as well of Carl Jung and Alfred Adler, his colleagues and successors, analyzed their dreams in psychotherapy sessions.

That gave me an idea. As soon as I was on the Clomipramine, I started having dreams in my sleep. Every night when the dream was finished, I immediately woke up and wrote down the details of the dream. At weekly group therapy sessions, I read out the stories of my dreams.

My dreams centered around episodes that I was involved in. I can only remember three of them. During this time I was studying political science at York University's Atkinson College. In one dream, I saw Robert Stanfield, a onetime leader of the Conservative Party. I remember Dr. Fenigstein asking me, "was he in his underwear?" referring to the Stanfield undergarments business. In another dream, I was being eaten by sharks. In a third dream, I was a baby in the middle of a circle of babies, who were singing, "Debbie the little flower girl."

In the group therapy sessions I was determined to get my symptoms under control. I insisted on working on my dreams at every session, often without consideration for the other group members who had their own problems. For this, I was considered to be aggressive and insensitive.

Discussing my dreams helped me to find a sense of self. Dr. Fenigstein agreed with the idea of analysing my dreams. He said, "You have to find yourself as well as learning to control your obsessive compulsive disorder. Whatever goals my patients have set themselves for therapy, in the end they all want to find themselves."

My dreams were only the beginning. I had to learn to relax completely and think of nothing consciously in order to unlock the secret of my unconscious mind. I was not able to do this until sometime later. Dr. Frank Cashman added the Lorazepam to my medication and started my sessions with his students and I began the behavioural therapy exercises from the Obsessive Compulsive Disorder Support Group which helped me to bring my symptoms under control so that I could relax and contemplate.

My mother was thankful that I finally knew what was wrong with me. A few psychiatrists in the

United States, including Dr. Michael Jenike, had collaborated on a landmark study of obsessive compulsive disorder, <u>Obsessive Compulsive Disorder Theory and Management</u>. Another psychiatrist, Dr. Judith Rapoport, had written a book entitled <u>The Boy Who Couldn't Stop Washing</u>. My mother found out about these books. She was able to interloan both books from the University of Toronto Medical Sciences Library through her hospital library. According to Dr. Jenike and Dr. Rapoport, the largest part of behaviour therapy is performing actions that the obsessive compulsive disorder sufferer is afraid to perform. That way the obsessive compulsive disorder sufferer discovers that his or her phobias are groundless.

My mother discovered through the books that medication alone would not bring my obsessive compulsive disorder under control. To combat obsessive compulsive disorder symptoms I also had to employ behavioural therapy. Behavioural therapy involved exercises to eliminate checking and repetition. It also involved using thought before action and speech to eliminate inappropriate and compulsive behaviour. From the books we found out about the Obsessive Compulsive Disorder Foundation that was based in Boston, Massachusetts. We joined the foundation and we received a monthly newsletter that contained exercises in behaviour therapy that I could practice at home.

My mother also read a number of articles in the Toronto Star which introduced readers to obsessive compulsive disorder. These articles are:

"The compulsion that won't go away", by Sheryl Ubelacker, Toronto Star, Friday, January 6, 1989, p. D1

"Self-help group for the obsessed set up in Toronto", by Sheryl Ubelacker, Toronto Star, Friday, January 6, 1989, p. D4

"Cause of mental illness could be biological", by Sheryl Ubelacker, Toronto Star, Friday, January 6, 1989, p. D4

From the same Toronto Star article which introduced readers to obsessive compulsive disorder, my mother and I learned of an obsessive compulsive disorder support group, the Toronto Support Group. It was not a therapy group. The Toronto Support Group allowed obsessive compulsive disorder sufferers to meet each other for support and share experiences. A telephone number to contact was listed in the newspaper article. I telephoned this number and learned that this group met every week in members' homes. I was immediately accepted. I told the other members that I was in group therapy with Dr. Fenigstein. My mother allowed the group to meet in our home when my turn came. Some of the other members of the group were patients of Dr. Frank Cashman, who at that time practiced at the Clark Institute of Psychiatry. Dr. Cashman and his colleague, Dr. Richard Swinson, also at the Clarke institute, were the only two psychiatrists in Toronto practicing exclusively in the area of obsessive compulsive disorder. I attended the obsessive compulsive disorder support group for two years

My therapy sessions with Dr. Fenigstein ended when he died. The group therapy sessions with the social workers, lasted six years, and also ended when he died. During this period when I was attending the group therapy sessions and the Toronto Support Group I went back to York University and studied at Atkinson College to complete my fourth year in political science and went to the University of Toronto where I completed a Master of Library Science degree (M.L.S.). During this time at Atkinson College I had a part-time job delivering as mail for Canada Post.

Intensive Therapy With Dr. Cashman

My family doctor, Dr. Bell, referred me to Dr. Frank Cashman, one of the few psychiatrists in Canada who specialized in obsessive compulsive disorder. At my first appointment with Dr. Cashman, I filled out a questionnaire outlining my obsessive compulsive disorder symptoms. I said to him, "I found out about you from the Toronto Support Group and then got a reference from Dr. Bell to see you. My mother and I belong to the Obsessive Compulsive Disorder Foundation in Massachusetts, and we get the monthly newsletter that outlines their behaviour therapy exercises. I was doing very well in my therapy with Dr. Henry Fenigstein at the North York Psychotherapy Clinic, and his sudden death left me in the lurch. I miss the group therapy."

All of my information he entered into his computer. Then he proceeded with what he had to say.

Dr. Cashman increased me from two to five 50mg pills of Clomipramine per day and added 2mg of Lorazepam to my medication per day. He said, "Your brain is unable to facilitate the use of serotonin by itself because you have no natural serotonin. The Lorazepam will enable you're your brain to process the serotonin and you will be able to control your symptoms."

He also said, "You are a very intelligent and sophisticated person, and these qualities will show once you are under control. You are also intellectually mature as a result of your history-oriented courses at the University of Toronto. You just need to mature emotionally and you will."

Thanks to the addition of Lorazepam, my symptoms finally were beginning to get under control. I told Dr. Cashman that I missed my therapy with Dr. Fenigstein. Dr. Cashman offered me alternative therapy.

Dr. Cashman suggested that I try yoga and transcendental meditation. Yoga required that I sit like a pretzel, which I was to clumsy to do, and transcendental meditation required attending classes, which I was not prepared to do.

"I don't do group therapy," he said, "but I can offer you something similar. I teach psychiatric residents at the University of Toronto. Would you like

to meet them? You can be a guinea pig in their classes.
They will ask you questions and you will answer them.
You will benefit. They in-turn will benefit from meeting
you. Most obsessive compulsive disorder sufferers are
very mentally disabled, but a few are very intelligent,
like you, and driven to accomplish, like you and well
educated, like you. Would you like to give their classes
a try?

I agreed to meet his students. I found talking to
them extremely helpful. At my first class, I told his
students, "The dogs of OCD come across me and burn
my brain, so that I cannot think straight."

Dr. Cashman, who was present, said to his
students, "We have to get Debbie to the point where the
dogs of OCD leave her alone and stay away."

Well, the classes with his students saved my
sanity. Slowly between the Clomipramine and
Lorazepam and my sessions with his students, my
symptoms finally got pretty well under control. I saw
Dr. Cashman twice a week for six months and then once
a month for ten years.

Before I stopped seeing Dr. Cashman I was able
to reduce my Clomipramine from five 50 mg pills per
day to four 50mg pills per day. The Lorazepam stayed
the same at 2 mg per day. After I stopped seeing Dr.
Cashman I was able to reduce the Clomipramine to
three 50 mg pills per day and reduce the Lorazepam to

1 mg per day. This is the level that I have been on for years now.

Behaviour Therapy

The Obsessive Compulsive Disorder Foundation sent me exercises in behaviour therapy that I could perform at home. I performed this type of therapy during the time I saw both Dr. Fenigstein and Dr. Cashman.

Behaviour therapy involves situations in which the obsessive compulsive disorder sufferer performs a task like locking a door. The person feels compelled to check if the door is locked. The therapist, or in this case, my mother prevents the person from checking the locked door, and switches the person away to perform a different task. Eventually the person remembers that he or she locked the door, and the compulsion disappears.

A person who suffers from obsessive compulsive disorder is also afraid of performing certain tasks or going to certain places out of fear that he or she will harm themselves or somebody else. Behaviour therapy involves performing the otherwise avoided tasks or going to the place that he or she has been otherwise avoiding and discovering that there was nothing to be afraid of.

Another obsessive compulsive disorder compulsion is to be a clock watcher. Clock watching is done in situations where the person is performing a task that takes time or attending an event. The person is afraid that the task will take all day or all night to perform because they are so slow. The person is also afraid that the event will last all day or all night. Behaviour therapy involved forcing the person to completely focus on the task at hand and performing it in a reasonable time period. It also involves forcing the person to concentrate on the event that they are attending and finding that it ends within an hour or a couple of hours. Clock watching tends to end with the realization that the person will finish the task and that the event will end, otherwise all workers will get fed up doing the work or the audience watching the event will be bored.

Another symptom of obsessive compulsive disorder is impatience. The person is unable to walk or relax or be patient. Behaviour therapy involves forcing the person to relax and be patient and enjoy doing tasks, taking walks, and watching evens as they go through life.

Rigidity is a symptom of obsessive compulsive disorder. The person is rigid when they perform the same routine day after day after day and cannot change. It also involves making only friends of the same ethnic group or who have the same personality as the person. Behaviour therapy means that the person learns to befriend all different kinds of people and changes their daily or weekly or monthly routine.

Rigidity is necessary when taking pills or when it means not driving after drinking liquor. But in most circumstances the person does not have to be rigid about their routine. Most people do not care if the other people they meet come from a similar or a different background and are open to meeting people from all walks of life.

Checking is a symptom of obsessive compulsive disorder. Behaviour therapy teaches the person to avoid checking something over and over again. A person may check multiple times that they have done something such as locking the door. The fact that a person needs to continually check that something has been done indicates a lack of confidence and that they are unsure of themselves. It is all right to check something once to be sure but when the person starts checking repeatedly then there is a problem. The person has to be instilled with a sense of confidence that they actually did things right the first time. Behaviour therapy allows the person to check once but when they finish they are pulled away. Eventually the person remembers that they did check.

Repetition is a symptom of obsessive compulsive disorder. Behaviour therapy teaches the person to avoid saying the same thing, asking the same question, or doing the same thing over and over again. The fact that a person needs to continually repeat indicates a lack of confidence and that they are unsure of themselves. The person has to be instilled with a sense of confidence that they said or did things right the first time and that there is no need to repeat them. Behaviour therapy means that if the person says or does something more than once they are cut off from saying or doing it again by the therapist.

Another symptom of obsessive compulsive disorder is keeping lists. Behaviour therapy teaches people not to keep lists that have no real purpose. It is all right to keep lists if they have a purpose such as accounting lists of money spent, shopping lists, lists of contact information for friends and relatives, lists of medications, other purposeful lists. But keeping lists becomes dangerous when the person starts keeping lists of absolutely everything in their life as well as lists of absolutely useless information. This information often has nothing to do with them and plays no part in their life. Behaviour therapy teaches the person to destroy the needless lists.

Another symptom of obsessive compulsive disorder is inappropriate sexual urges. The person can feel like having sex with the wrong people, such as co-workers, bosses, married people, a caregiver, or a therapist. When I was in the Obsessive Compulsive Disorder Support Group, I met a few men who were taking Clomipramine and Lorazepam. All of the men told the group that the Clomipramine controlled their sexual urges to the point that they were impotent. I remember feeling sorry for these men because I believe that appropriate sexual activity is one of life's most enjoyable activities.

Obsessive compulsive disorder can be boiled down to severe anxiety. Severe anxiety can lead the person to mutilate their bodies, destroy their minds by taking narcotic drugs, or spend whole days worrying. In extreme cases, obsessive compulsive disorder can lead the person to commit suicide. For many extreme cases, the psychiatrist has to have the person hospitalized in order to prevent them from destroying themselves. I feel thankful that I am able to perform behaviour therapy exercises on myself with help from Glen, or I would have to be hospitalized. I am also happy that before my marriage, I was able to do the exercises with my mother. Otherwise, instead of studying and writing, I could have spent years in a psychiatric institution.

Therapy Outline

The following is the approximate order in which I had therapy:

<u>No. 1:</u> Dr. Irving Zelcer – Family Physician – spoke to him but he said all OHIP psychiatrists were booked up

<u>No. 2</u> Helen Sugar – Social Worker Jewish Family and Child Services

No. 3 Heather McPherson – Social Worker Bayview Avenue Therapy Centre

No. 4 Dr. William Bell – Family Physician – referred me to Dr. Brody

No. 5 Dr. Brody – Psychiatrist – referred me to Dr. Henry Fenigstein

No. 6 Dr. Skain – Gynecologist – gave me some helpful advice about OCD

No.7 Dr. Henry Fenigstein – Psychiatrist North York Psychotherapy Centre

No. 8 Group Therapy Sessions with Social Workers who worked for Dr. Henry Fenigstein

No. 9 Books on psychology given to me in private appointments with Dr. Henry Fenigstein – reading the books and writing essays on them

No. 10 Obsessive Compulsive Disorder Foundation - joining and doing the behaviour therapy lessons which they sent me – these were done during the time I saw Dr. Fenigstein and Dr. Cashman

No. 11 Reading books on psychology and obsessive compulsive disorder – these were read during the time that I saw Dr. Fenigstein

No. 12   Dr. William Bell – Family Physician – referred me to Dr. Frank Cashman after Dr. Fenigstein died

No. 13   Toronto Support Group which met at members' homes

No. 14   Dr. Frank Cashman – Psychiatrist Specializing in Obsessive compulsive Disorder – worked at Clarke Institute of Psychiatry, Wellesley Hospital, and St. Michael's Hospital

No. 15   Sessions with Psychiatric Students of Dr. Frank Cashman

No. 16   Dr. Lauren Torbin – Family Doctor – my family doctor for a time who also did psychotherapy sessions; I saw her for a while with Glen shortly before and for a time after we were married

Obsessive Compulsive Disorder Symptoms

Symptoms of obsessive compulsive disorder vary from person to person. Mine were:

No. 1 Checking: Checking and rechecking things I had done

No. 2 Repeating: Repeating over and over things I had done and said

No. 3 Lists: Keeping multiple lists of both useful and useless information

No. 4 Reading and writing too slowly. I did work in school and university very slowly, e.g. class work, assignments, tests, and exams

No. 5 Inability to concentrate. I was unable to keep my mind on something for very long and got bored easily. I often had a hard time sitting through lectures. Although I read history, historical fiction, and literature beyond my years, I was unable to write summaries or make notes on what I read.

No. 6 Performing tasks too slowly. I was unable to do routine jobs in offices.

No. 7 Rigidity: Things had to be done in a certain way. Things had to be placed in a certain way. Things had to be done at a certain time. Things have to be said in a certain way. Opinions and views different than my own were not tolerated.

No. 8 Biting my nails.

No. 9 Mutilating my fingers and my skin.

No. 10 Taking what people said literally.

No. 11 Talking to myself. I used to whisper stories to myself.

No. 12 Writing on the air with my index finger or a pen.

No. 13 Staring at people and making people uncomfortable to be around me.

No. 14 Irrational thoughts.

No. 15 Impatience, clock-watching, and rushing.

No. 16 Anxiety: Anticipating and worrying about situations that either have not happened, will not happen, could not happen, or have happened.

No. 17 Fear of saying something wrong, not saying something just right, or leaving out details of what I said.

No. 18 Repeatedly seeking reassurance. This involved asking if I had done something right or if I had done something wrong or about something I had heard or seen. This was, in other words, seeking continual confirmation.

Other symptoms which I did not have and which should be mentioned are:

No. 19 Hoarding. Hoarders are people who keep everything whether they need it or not and whether it is valuable or not. Most often it is things that they do not need and which have no value other than perhaps a nostalgic or sentimental value. Hoarders tend to let their possessions take them and their lives over. They can be inundated with material possessions to the point where it can cost them their family, their friends, their jobs, money, and their home. Their homes often become filled with wall to wall possessions to the point where there is no place to move and where it becomes a fire and a health hazard. Hoarding is a very dangerous form of obsessive compulsive disorder and one that needs to be stopped in its tracks before it gets out of hand.

No. 20 Extreme cleanliness. People with this compulsion are afraid of germs and may wash themselves and everything around them repeatedly.

 No. 21 Watching the weather continuously. Some people worry too much about the weather and listen and watch news about the weather too much. At the Hamilton Obsessive Compulsive Disorder Support Group the group was told that for these people their entire lives and what they do can revolve around the weather and that they have fears of what the weather may be. They may be afraid to leave their homes because of a weather report and isolate themselves. The group was told that the Weather Network was the worst thing for people with this type of obsessive compulsive disorder as they would spend the whole day watching and worrying about the weather. The repetition factor is also involved as the weather station keeps repeating basically the same things over and over again all day.

<u>No. 22</u> Fanaticism. This involves extreme belief in a doctrine or philosophy which may be environmental, political, social, or religious. The belief can control the person's whole life and all his relationships.

<u>Singles Groups, Dating, and Therapy</u>

During my high school years in Montreal both television shows and teen magazines extolled the virtues of teenagers having parties with friends and dating. My classmates were heavily into the teenaged dating scene and always fixed each other up with dates. Because I had no friends, I was left out of the big social whirl. As I passed my fifteenth and sixteenth birthdays, friendless and boy friendless, I was afraid that I was missing out on a wonderful world of fun.

"I am sixteen years old," I complained to my mother during the summer that I was sixteen, "and I have never had a date."

My mother answered, "It's too bad you are the first child in our family. Girls your age meet dating partners either through older siblings or through girlfriends. You have neither. Also, you do not belong to a crowd. Girls who move in crowds of boys and girls date sooner than girls who don't belong to a crowd."

I think that the crowning humiliation of my high school years in Montreal was being forced to miss my graduation prom because I had no date.

Among the obsessive compulsive disorder symptoms that surfaced during my sixteenth summer were uncontrollable sexual urges. Because I had no dates, I was worried that I would never be able to have sex. For some people sex outside of marriage is always considered socially unacceptable although it has always occurred and is now more socially acceptable by most people.

I remember at the time watching a movie on television starring Shirley Jones as the teacher in a special school for pregnant teenagers. A sign of obsessive compulsive disorder was that I wanted to be like those girls.

"When I see movies like this one, "I told my mother, "I am reminded that I have never had a date or a boyfriend."

"If you had a boyfriend," my mother asked me, "would you be having sexual intercourse with him?"

"Yes, I would." I answered.

After we moved to Toronto, my social life picked up. When a new friend at MacKenzie Collegiate fixed me up with a blind date, my very first date, my mother was happy for me.

"It looks like we have come to a nice place," she said. "I think it is disgusting that in the whole City of Montreal you could not find a date for your high school graduation."

From that first date, I went on to have many more dates in both Grade 13 and throughout the years I spent at York University. At York, I met nice fellows both on <u>Excalibur</u> and in an ethnic organization to which I belonged.

My girlfriends from MacKenzie Collegiate and York University all got married right out of university. As I attended weddings, my obsessive compulsive disorder symptoms manifested themselves in a fear that I would never get married. I began a frenzied social life in which I joined singles groups and encouraged fellows whom I met to take my telephone number and call me for dates.

My desire to get married superseded other needs, such as holding down a job. Because we did not know about the obsessive compulsive disorder, my mother worried that my performance on my jobs was caused by laziness and an abnormal desire to get married.

"You don't have any desire to do your work well," she accused me.

"The reason I don't care about my work is that I feel that it is pointless because I can't get married." I answered.

"Is it pointless to do a good job just because you are not married?" my mother asked. "You are wasting your life. You can't hold down a job because you don't take pride in your work. All that you care about is running around with guys."

When I was in therapy with the social worker, Helen Sugar, I told her that everyone I knew was getting married and I was afraid I would be left out.

She answered, "Would it be so terrible if you did not marry? There was a stigma attached to being single. For women, anything in pants was considered better than being not married. That stigma has now largely ceased, but a lot of parents still want their daughters to get married. That is why the girls you knew got married right out of university. Their parents pushed it. That doesn't mean you have to be a copycat and marry anything in pants because they did."

My complex about being single persisted into my therapy with the social worker Heather McPherson. Heather told me flat out, "As a married woman you would have problems because you do not have a sense of self."

"What is a sense of self?" I asked her.

"A sense of self means that you know how you want to live your life as opposed to copying what other women are doing with their lives." she said.

I lost my complex about being single when I first entered Dr. Fenigstein's therapy groups. Before I met Elaine, I met a lot of divorced women who had been pushed into young marriages by their parents. Consequently, these women were unhappy and they had children to support.

After I was on Clomipramine, I began to be thankful that I had not married. I realized that wanting to be married so much was the result of uncontrolled obsessive compulsive disorder.

During the course of intensive therapy, I realized that to be happy in a marriage you have to be in love with your spouse. I remember asking both Dr. Fenigstein and Dr. Cashman, "How do you know when you are in love?" Dr. Fenigstein recommended that I read Erich Fromm's The Art of Loving. I read the book, but I still had no yardstick for measuring true love. Dr. Cashman told me, "Debbie, I don't really know. I just know that when you are in love, you know it."

Before I met Glen I went to a lot of singles events and singles groups both at university and when I was working. I was looking for guys of the same ethnic group as me. This idea had been ingrained in me by my mother. I was also looking for guys who were university educated and had professions. My shopping list for a husband consisted of those factors. Some of the ones I met had bad personality problems and psychiatric problems of their own showing that being of the same ethnic group as me, having a university education, and having a profession does not guarantee that the person has a likeable personality or is mentally stable. Also my obsessive compulsive disorder symptoms such as the ones I previously listed were obvious and were a turnoff for the ones whom I liked and who were normal. I do not want to go into specific details about my past dates because Glen does not want to read about them and because I do not want to offend anybody.

More Singles Groups, Dating and Therapy

It was while I was in therapy with Helen Sugar at Jewish Family and Child Services at Jewish Family and Child Services that my mother decided to try to marry me off. One of her cousins, Lawrence Simons and his wife, Rose Simons, married off their two daughters, Norma and Leah. Both Norma and Leah had babies right away, making Lawrence and Rose grandparents. At the same time, my mother had two friends Jasmine and her husband Scott; and Fay and her husband Moti. Each couple married off two children: Brandon and Sharon, and Roberta and Jane. All four children produced babies right away, thereby making their parents grandparents.

Whenever my mother got together with her cousins, Lawrence and Rose, and with her friends, Jasmine and Fay, conversation would involve around marriages, pregnancies, and grandchildren. Inevitably, Lawrence, Rose, Jasmine, and Fay asked my mother, "When is Debbie going to get married and make you a grandmother?" My mother answered defensively, "Debbie is fussy. She doesn't want to marry just anybody. She wants to marry somebody fancy. She also tells Maurice and me that she doesn't want children.

"She doesn't want to get married and have children?" asked Lawrence, Rose, Jasmine, and Fay in disbelief. "What type of Jewish girl does not want to get married or have children?"

One evening after her cousin and friends left, my mother said to my father, "Why doesn't Debbie just settle down, get married, and have children, like other Jewish women? Why do we have to worry about her?"

My father answered, "If Debbie feels that she doesn't want to get married, that's her choice."

"She would get married if she met the right person," my mother persisted. "To bad we don't know anybody who can fix her up with a blind date."

"She's very fussy," my father answered. "Even if she was fixed up with a blind date, she might not like him."

At this time, I was dating a fellow named Harold Fineberg. He was an M.B.A. graduate who worked as a systems analyst for Sears. He was saving his money for marriage, and begrudged every cent that he spent on me. He also did not like that I had been terminated from five jobs, and kept hoping that I would finally get a permanent job. He finally dumped me because I was jobless.

I went back to singles dances and had a few dates, but the fellows did not treat me with respect, so I did not bother encouraging them to call me for a second date. One fellow, named Jeff, called me a nice broad. I sent him away.

My mother sat me down and told me that I should have treated the "nice broad" phrase as a joke.

"I want you to get married and I want grandchildren," she said. "It is better to be married than single, and you should look bloody hard and not just terminate a relationship without a second thought."

At my next session with Helen Sugar, I told her of my mother's ambition to marry me off and see to it that I made her a grandmother.

Helen said, "Ask your mother if she is so eager for you to get married, what you will get out of a loveless marriage?"

When I got home and asked my mother this question, she got angry and yelled at me, "Who is filling your head with this crap?"

I answered, "Helen at Jewish Family and Child Services."

"Is Helen married or single?" my mother asked.

I answered, "Helen is single."

My mother said to me, "You call up Jewish Family and Child Services and tell them that you want to switch to a married social worker."

"Why?" I asked my mother.

"Because a married social worker will give you a more realistic view of marriage," my mother answered. "I am telling you that I have been married for twenty-six years and my experience is that a woman gets zero out of marriage."

In an effort to clam up my mother, I reluctantly called up Jewish Family and Child Services. When I told them that I wanted to switch to a married social worker, they asked me, "Why?" When I told them I was enquiring at my mother's request, they flatly refused. They told me that they do not base a social worker's qualifications on her marital status.

At my next appointment, Helen blasted me for basing her competence as a social worker on her marital status.

"At the age of 25," she said, "you should be asking your mother's permission to see me. I think that your mother's assessment of a woman's role in marriage is hilarious and at the same time, it is very, very, sad. I know women who have been married thirty years, and they have beautiful fulfilling marriages."

After my father's death, my mother decided that what she wanted most was to see her children married and to have a house full of grandchildren. She gave me what she thought was a strategy to persuade a man to propose. As it happened, I dated two fellows who, after our initial dates, requested that I phone them.

One of my boyfriends, Donald Dicks, said to me, "Debbie, I get busy working in my job and sometimes I forget about you. If you want to go out with me, feel free to call me and set it up. If you see in the newspaper a movie or a play that you want to see, call me and we will set it up together."

The first time that I phoned Donald, my mother made me hang up the phone. "Don't you dare call up a guy for a date," she yelled at me. You make him call you and make him marry you when he asks you for sex. If you insist that you don't put out unless you are married, he will have to come across."

Malcolm Denver, my other boyfriend, also requested that I phone him if I wanted to go out on a date, because he happened to be a busy hairdresser. Well I gave in to my mother's wish and did not phone Donald or Malcolm. As a result, the relationships went nowhere. When I told my mother that the relationships terminated because of her insistence that I not phone them, she laughed at me. "Those fellows didn't really love you," she said. 'Otherwise they would have phoned you. Don't worry, the right fellow will do all the phoning."

One more relationship went sour because I refused my boyfriend's request to phone him. Then I met Glen. We fell in love right away. When Glen requested that I telephone him, I did not want to lose him, too. So, to my mother's chagrin, I telephoned him. My mother accused me of chasing him like a tramp, but I ignored her. Because I followed my heart, and not my mother's wishes, we married.

Glen and I

Glen grew up in the Forest Hill neighbourhood of Toronto. His parents followed his father's legal career and moved to Hamilton. We first met after I graduated from the University of Toronto and was looking for a job as a librarian. Glen was a graduate of McMaster University, University of Western Ontario, and University of Waterloo. He had degrees in Sociology, Political Science, Library Science, and Recreation and Leisure. Glen was teaching part-time in the Humanities and Social Sciences Department at Mohawk College in Hamilton after finishing graduate school when I met him.

We met in a singles bowling group in Toronto. The group met every Sunday. When we met, I told him that I was looking for a full-time job as a librarian. Glen said to me, "I have a Master's Degree in Library Science from the University of Western Ontario and I have not been able to find a job in a library." We talked for quite a while and we found that we had many interests in common.

On the following Sunday, Glen asked me for my telephone number and said that he would call me during the week. He called during the week and on the Saturday, I believe, we went on our first date to the Royal Ontario Museum. We saw each other regularly after that.

I first told Glen that I had obsessive compulsive disorder some time later into our relationship. I'm not exactly sure when, but I believe, it was within a couple of months after we met. I told him what obsessive compulsive disorder was, how I was being treated, and what the symptoms were. I was worried that he would leave me because of it. He said that he saw no detectable symptoms and wanted us to stay together. We have been together ever since.

Glen said that he had experienced symptoms that may be classified as obsessive compulsive disorder since he was a child but that they were not consistent and would disappear for long periods at a time and then return and disappear again.

When we had been together about a year when Penguin Books ran a contest in which the participants had to look at classic literature and write down the first lines of various classics. We submitted the first lines but never heard from them. From that Glen and I got the idea of compiling an index of famous first lines from literature as a reference book. We had seen in the bookstores indexes of last lines of books and thought naively that this index would be a great idea as it had not been done before.

The result was that we compulsively went to Toronto Reference Library, North York Central Library, some of the smaller Toronto Library branches, Hamilton Public Library, and the University of Toronto and York University Libraries to write down first lines and then put them by author in alphabetical order and put them on a computer database. We were doing this compulsively in our spare time for about two years. That is not to say that we did not do other things. We certainly did many other things. And Glen had just got his job as an Estate Researcher with the Public Guardian and Trustee, so these first lines were done between everything else.

But the way we did the first lines was compulsive. We were going all out, so to speak, to find and complete the first lines of the books by famous writers. We had these far-fetched ideas that we were doing some great reference book that the publishers would jump at. We made inquiries to a number of publishers and a couple of them asked us to send them excerpts of about twenty pages. They were rejected.

We stopped and realized that the entire idea was stupid and in fact, we were doing a type of obsessive compulsive disorder behaviour by keeping lists. Even if we were to consider doing this type of first line index what we should have done was to contact publishers first to see if they were in fact interested and if there was any demand for such a project. We were stupid and obsessive and the result was that we completely wasted any time that was spent on the entire project.

During our marriage I would say that I have had numerous problems with obsessive compulsive disorder symptoms and it is often a struggle to keep them controlled. I am doing my best and Glen is very understanding because he sometimes has obsessive compulsive disorder symptoms too. I would say that the only four obsessive compulsive disorder symptoms that I still have a problem with are (1) checking (2) repeating (3) impatience, clock-watching, and rushing (4) anxiety. I do my best to control them but I have times, usually short, when I lose control. I have also developed weather related OCD symptoms. This involves checking the weather a lot on the Weather Network. I tend to worry about the weather especially if they say it is going to rain and there could be thunderstorms.

After Library School and Beyond

I never did get a paying job in a library. I worked part-time for a while as a volunteer librarian at a Toronto school library and worked for a number of years as a part-time volunteer librarian in the Canadiana Room at North York Central Library. I also served for a year on the Toronto Reference Library Board.

I married and moved to Hamilton as was discussed previously. I took courses and received diplomas from the Canadian Securities Institute. There were, however, no jobs available. I was on the Mayor's Advisory Committee For Persons With Disabilities for one year. I was on the Hamilton Historical Board for 4 years and had articles published in their newsletter, HistoriCity. I am now writing poems and short stories and am a member of three poetry societies: Hamilton Poetry Centre, Tower Poetry Society, and the Ontario Poetry Society. Many of my poems have been published. I have also been doing some public poetry readings in association with the poetry societies. I am now, however, more interested in writing stories. Many of the short stories that I have written have also been published. So I now have a resume of poetry and story literary publications. I am regularly attending author, literary, poetry, and writing related events, lectures, and workshops many of them offered by Hamilton Public Library. I attend the yearly Word On The Street Book Festival in Toronto and would highly recommend it for all things book, magazine, digital publishing, and literary related.

Becoming involved with different groups and organizations as well as writing and reading is a very effective form of behaviour therapy because it keeps my mind active and does not allow me to dwell on nonsense. I am an avid reader and read the classics of literature as well as more contemporary novels. I especially enjoy historical fiction. I also read biography, history, and graphic novels.

Controlling my obsessive compulsive disorder takes every minute of my existence. I still tend to check, repeat, be impatient, and have anxiety at times. Not all the time but I go through periods, usually not long, where I do.

I will often repeat the same thing to Glen or ask him a question multiple times. I have also found myself doing it to other people at times. I am often impatient when Glen and I go somewhere and I tend to get restless or want to leave even though I know there is no reason to and that I wanted to come in the first place. I get impatient with Glen when we are in bookstores (Coles, Chapters, Indigo) if he starts looking at a book. He lets me look at whatever I want for as look as I want and never says anything. But, not all the time, but sometimes, I keep going at him to put the book down and grilling him about why he is looking at the book. I also tend to do that to him at times when he is working on the computer. I also tend to grill and question him about basically things that aren't even worth talking about. I know it is wrong and that I have got to control it.

I still have anxiety about things such as the weather, health, and eating. I worry about the weather sometimes and whether there will be precipitation. I have to watch what I eat for health reasons. There is a history of diabetes in the family so I have to be very careful about what I eat. As a result of this I tend to eat at certain times quite rigidly, perhaps too rigidly. I also have to avoid foods with cholesterol and trans-fat. In 2010, I went for a complete physical to a private medical clinic in Toronto. The physical examination cost was very expensive, which Glen paid for, but you got all sorts of tests, both blood tests and other tests, that are not routinely given by physicians for a physical who are in OHIP. You get over fifty blood tests and the results come back by the end of your visit which is about six hours. The results of some of the other tests will also be ready at the end of the visit while the results of others will be ready within a week. I was already on medication for high blood pressure when I went for the physical. They found a urinary tract infection, high cholesterol, and a bicuspid aorta. Well, they probably saved my life.

I was put on antibiotics for the infection which cleared up. My family doctor, Dr. M. Z., after seeing these results sent me to a specialist, Dr. G. C., who put me on cholesterol medication. Along with watching my diet, which is vegetarian, this put my cholesterol back to normal. The bicuspid aorta is stable and will be fine as long as I take care of myself. I just have to watch myself, eat right, walk, take my medications, and I will be healthy. I attend Dr. G. C.'s health lectures and Sobeys (which is a large supermarket in Ancaster) health classes and workshops which are run by a registered dietician. Part of my path to good health is also controlling my obsessive compulsive disorder and keeping relaxed and not stressing myself about nonsense.

I also tend to worry that Glen will not eat. He is thin and I am concerned that he does not eat enough, particularly by the fact that his mother starved herself. He says that that he eats fine and what he is able to and that I am worrying for nothing. He is probably right.

In the summer, and I know that it is silly, but I still at times tend to worry that thunderstorms will cause a power failure. Our hydro polls are underground, so there is no danger of thunder or lightening hitting a hydro pole. We have actually only had a few power outages. Possibly lightning struck the above ground transformer. Before last winter, 2013 – 2014, I never even thought about snow. I drove our car all over Hamilton and the surrounding area. After the horrendous ice storm, the roads were thick with ice for a few months. When Glen and I drove anywhere, the car would skid and slide. I was always afraid after the ice storm of causing or getting into an accident. Well, the past winter of 2014 – 2015 saw normal snow falls. I panicked every time we went anywhere, but my fears were groundless. Wherever I drove, the driving was normal. But I still panic, after the ice storm, when, freezing rain is in the weather forecast. But in Hamilton this year we have seen very little freezing rain. I think that I have this basically under control and while the idea may go through my mind at times, I know that it is ridiculous, and to just ignore it.

I find that I still dwell a lot on the past both in my mind and verbally. I tend to think and talk repeated about the way I was treated by my family, other people, and different events and places. Memories tend to be both pleasant and unpleasant and I tend to sometimes go over at nauseum both types.

A number of years ago I read a book on obsessive compulsive disorder which I can recommend as it can help the sufferer work through his or her problem with exercises. The book is <u>The OCD Workbook: Your Guide to Breaking Free From Obsessive-Compulsive Disorder</u> by Bruce M. Hyman and Cherry Patrick, Oakland, California: New Harbinger Publications, 2005.

I have not mentioned much about my brother Bradley in this memoir. He used to tease me a lot about my behaviour when I was growing up and afterwards. He now says that he is very sorry for that because he didn't understand what was wrong with me. He did not understand what obsessive compulsive disorder was and was so involved with school, work, and his own life that he didn't have the time to pay attention to my problems. This is something that he deeply regrets.

I think that's all that I have to say for now. I think that you must from reading this memoir now have an idea about what obsessive compulsive disorder is, what it's symptoms are, and how it can be treated. Most important, if you or someone whom you know has symptoms of obsessive compulsive disorder do not ignore them. Do research and ask your doctor for help.

Poetry

I have been writing short stories and poetry and am a member of a number of poetry groups. I have written a number of poems which relate to my experiences with obsessive compulsive disorder.

Elaine

I met Elaine in group therapy,
and connected with her immediately.
Elaine was strange,
and couldn't sit still,
She walked in and out of the room,

back and forth, back and forth.
She couldn't hold a job because her work was slow,
and was fired from every job.
She was on medication for a psychiatric disorder,
that I has never heard of.
She was recommended for therapy by her doctor,
and told her story in group therapy.
She had problems communicating with people,
and did not come across logically.
She had the same symptoms as I do,
and through her I found out,
all about my obsessive compulsive disorder.

Obsessive Compulsive Disorder

My head feels like it is on fire,
when I do not take my medication.
I pace the floor all night,
when I do not take my medication.
My brain feels like it will explode,
when I do not take my medication.
I cannot control my thought processes,
when I do not take my medication.
My feelings are easily hurt,
when I do not take my medication.
My face looks strained,
when I do not take my medication.
Because I want to look, sound, and feel
good all the time,
I take my medication.

The following two poems describes the atmosphere in which I grew up:

Growing Up in Cote St. Luc

The money flowed like champagne,
at a New Year's Eve party.
Our neighbours were rich and brassy-sassy-smarty.

My classmates talked incessantly,
about their father's new car,
their mother's new furniture and carpet,
and their basement wet bar.

Nouveau-riche people in Cote St. Luc,
wore expensive clothes and enough,
diamonds to make you puke.

My family did not belong in Cote St. Luc.
We ended up being there,
through a sheer fluke.
My parent bought a house,
they really did not want,
because the houses they really liked,
were already sold out,
and what was available was scant.

We wore shabby clothes,
because we were poor.
Poor enough that people stared,
when we walked out the door.

Cote St. Lucers saw spending money,
as a status symbol.
Municipal taxes were high,
but our neighbours did not tremble.
Public transportation,
did not go far,
but about this they cavalierly said,
"Everybody here has a car."
Making money was their god,
for they decorated lavish homes,
and took expensive trips abroad.
All doctors, lawyers, C.A.'s and engineers,
who associated with others,
whom they counted as their peers.

Of my childhood,
the happiest day,
was the day,
we moved away,
from Cote St. Luc – hurray!

A Sound Heard in Childhood

The sound that I most remember is of my parents
fighting.
They fought all the time.
Continually yelling and screaming.
Sometimes my mother would hit my father.
They fought about my brother and me.

Did my mother really want children?
I wondered because I remember things,
like her complaining about how she had to look after us.
They fought about my father's job.
She felt that he did not earn enough money.
Did she really want to be married to a wealthy man?
I wondered because I remember things,
like her always complaining about the way we lived.
Her voice was shrill and ugly.
She used to literally scream.
My father didn't take the shouting easily.
He used to fight back.
His screams were so loud,
you could hear them in other parts of the world.
My parents really went after each other,
like two armies fighting,
until one achieved victory.
My mother used to threaten to walk out,
and leave us two children to fend for ourselves.
I remember being afraid she would and wondering,
whether she would she carry out her threat?
If she did, what would we do without her?
How would I fend for myself?
What would I do?
It is a worry that haunted me throughout my childhood.
I still wonder today.
What would life have been if she had walked out?
It is a thought that repeats itself in my adulthood.

The following poem describes my fear of
thunderstorms:

Thunderstorms

My OCD makes me afraid,
Sometimes unreasonably afraid.
I am afraid of the weather,
I am terrified of thunderstorms,
The sky gets black as night,
and all the heavens break loose,
with thunder and lightning,
Like a wild beast shooting down from the sky,
thunder seems to crack the house into fragments,
of wood, glass, and concrete.
Lightning pierces the sky so bright,
that it looks like the middle of the day.
The storm makes the sky,
dark and bright simultaneously.
The electricity goes off,
and we are helpless without power.
My heart beats rapidly in fear,
and my head is spinning away so that,
the room rocks back and forth.
My legs feel like cotton batten,
and I wish the thunderstorm would end,
so that the power can be restored,
and we can get back to our normal activities.
Or, better still, may the meteorologist be wrong,
and the thunderstorm may not come at all.
Maybe I just have an exaggerated phobia,
but I am terrified of thunderstorms.
Driving is treacherous,
because lightning can crack the windows.

So it is a good precaution to stay home,
where there is shelter,
or drive carefully to a shopping mall,
until the power returns.
My stomach gurgles and I pace the floor.
I pace all through the house with anxiety,
Looking at the sky to see when,
the thunderstorm will end

The following poem describes my feelings about driving after the ice storm:

<u>After the Ice Storm</u>

After the ice storm,
the car was slip-sliding on the ice.
After the ice storm,
the roads were skating rinks.
After the nice storm,
The car was weaving and the tires were spinning.
After the ice storm,
the car won't stop when I pushed the brakes.
After the ice storm,
I was driving with feelings of deep apprehension.
After the ice storm,
the world was white and gaunt.
After the ice storm,
driving the car was dangerous.
New snow tires for the car,
let me drive safely,
after an ice storm.

The following humorous story happened during my summer job at the court house:

At The Court House

by

Deborah Eker

When I was a university student, I was able through my uncle to get summer jobs at the Court House in downtown Toronto. My uncle worked full-time for the Ontario government.

I worked for the Registrar of the Supreme Court of Ontario, whose office was responsible for divorce procedures. Decrees Absolute or divorce papers were issued by the Typist's Office for a person who wanted copies of the divorce papers. Orders for divorce papers took five working days to process.

I was borrowed from the Central Office for a few days to work in the Typist's Office. One of my customers was the male half of a couple who were getting married. The man was divorced and was remarrying. He demanded his Decree Absolute right away.

"I'm sorry, sir," I had to tell him, "but we require five working days to process your order for your divorce papers."

The gentleman, who was accompanied by his fiancée, blasted me, but left when she threatened to call her supervisor. I was busy with other work and I forgot about the incident.

At the end of the day, I went to the Central Office to sign out on her time sheet. Central Office was where plaintiffs and their lawyers presented their petitions for divorce to counter clerks and where the entire divorce procedure was initiated.

I told one of the counter clerks about the incident at the Typist's Office. "Some people don't take 'no' for an answer," I said as I signed out. "This fellow was enraged when I told him that he would have to wait five days for his Decree Absolute. And he is getting married again. I pity his poor wife."

One of the counter clerks, Gordon, spoke up.

"Gee", he said, "I wonder if that was the same dodo who came stomping in here, swearing at me, calling me every four-letter word in the book, banging on the counter and shouting, "I WANT MY DIVORCE PAPERS." A mismatch about to happen, I'm afraid."

Incidents like these made working at the Court House interesting.

A few days later, I went to work to find a heavy obnoxious odour in the air. So bad was this odour that people were covering their noses and waving fans in the air.

Finally around mid-morning, one of the clerks who worked directly for the Registrar started making a round of all the offices with the following request:

"Order from the Registrar. Would the person who hasn't changed his socks for two weeks please do so?"

This request fell on deaf ears. The obnoxious odour persisted all that day.